Bullying in Adulthood

D0060935

Peter Randall's first book, *Adult Bullying*, was one of the first books to examine the various situations in which adult bullying occurs, the forms it takes, and how it can be identified and dealt with more efficiently, particularly in workplace settings. Since that title was published, there has been more awareness of the extent of adult bullying.

In *Bullying in Adulthood: Assessing the Bullies and their Victims*, other aspects of the problem are examined, such as research and clinical issues, and in particular, assessment of bullies and victims and the background factors to such behaviour. This has become increasingly important as the problem begins to be appreciated and addressed within therapeutic, social and legal arenas. A number of strategies are suggested both for dealing with bullying and victim behaviour and for monitoring situations, for example by employers to see if problems improve. To assist in this process Peter Randall proposes a model of adult bullying which enables clinicians and human resources specialists to determine which factors are influential in individual cases. This book will appeal to practitioners and researchers in clinical/counselling psychology, counsellors, managers/human resources staff and social workers.

Peter Randall is Senior Research Fellow at the University of Hull where he continues to study bullying and other forms of interpersonal aggression. He is the author of *Adult Bullying: Perpetrators and Victims*.

Bullying in Adulthood

Assessing the bullies and their victims

Peter Randall

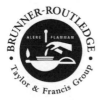

First published 2001 by Brunner Routledge
27 Church Road, Hove, East Sussex BN3 2FA

Simultaneously published in the USA and Canada
by Taylor & Francis Inc.
29 West 35th Street, New York, NY 10001

Brunner-Routledge is an imprint of the Taylor & Francis Group

Reprinted 2002

Typeset in Times by RefineCatch Limited, Bungay, Suffolk
Printed and bound in Great Britain by Biddles Ltd,
Guildford and King's Lynn
Cover design by Terry Foley

British Library Cataloguing in Publication Data
A catalogue record for this book is available from the British Library

Library of Congress Cataloging in Publication Data
Randall, Peter, 1948–
    Bullying in adulthood : assessing the bullies and their victims /
Peter Randall.
        p.   cm.
    Includes bibliographical references and index.
    1. Bullying.   2. Bullying in the workplace.   I. Title.
    BF637.B85 R37   2001
    650.1′3—dc21   2001035110

ISBN 0–415–23693–2 (hbk)
ISBN 0–415–23694–0 (pbk)

This book is dedicated to the memory of my friend
Mike Donohue whose compassionate work gave strength
to many victims.

Contents

Preface

It is an eloquent and tragic testimony to the power of adult bullying to cause severe psychological harm that concern about this subject has been burgeoning since the now sadly deceased Andrea Adams produced in 1992 her landmark book *Bullying at Work*. Since that time the acceptance of bullying as an adult as well as a child activity has led to a vast amount of research, formation of policies, legal actions and media attention.

The nature of this activity has inevitably emphasised its sensational and tragic aspects but careful research and clinical investigations have been gaining momentum and growing rapidly in the background of media portrayal. As a result, adult bullying is now increasingly well understood and the scientific research outcomes are filtering through to influence strategies at both the levels of protection and intervention. My own research into adult bullying at the clinical level has continued and has increasingly involved one-to-one work with perpetrators and victims. Much of this has arisen from employee assistance work but increasingly as part of a legal investigatory process informing subsequent proceedings.

I wished to take the published work a step further into the arena of practice by drawing together research and clinical studies to provide a first book on the assessment of bullies and victims in the context of the factors that cause them to act in the ways that they do. In part this is stimulated by the need to break down the excessive polarisation that exists at present. In essence, there is an overly simplistic assumption that victims are innocent people to whom bullying happens and bullies are undesirables who abuse others. Whereas this is often the case, clinical experience indicates that many victims bring into the workplace difficulties such as emotional 'unfinished business' which stimulate hostile responses. In other cases perpetrators may be shaped into their aggressive behaviour by workplace environments that reinforce hostile management or displacement behaviours. In addition, there may also be a rippling effect beyond the immediate workplace environment such that observers and family members may suffer secondary effects indirectly.

Assessments of perpetrators and victims are necessary not only from the viewpoint of prevention, intervention and dispute resolution, but also from the systemic platform of circular causality. This may be stated simply: dys-functional relationships promote bullying which creates further dysfunction. This book endeavours to explore these issues and show how they interact to produce a far-reaching disturbance of people's self-constructs and daily living.

For nearly thirty years I have studied and worked with human aggression taking the forms of physical child abuse, domestic violence, school bullying and workplace aggression. This has taught me that although the settings are very different the interpersonal factors are similar, the antecedents common and predictable. Adult bullying appears increasingly to me to be another form of human aggression but with more similarities than differences when compared with the others. The most common arena for its study is the workplace, and the high quality of empirical research provides detailed understanding of the factors that influence and perpetuate this behaviour. Empiricism, however, does not always enable understanding at the clinical level or of the degree of damage done to individuals. I hope that this book is a reasonable attempt to bridge the gap by bringing together the scientific study of adult bullying with the assessment of its psychopathological outcomes.

Acknowledgements

I acknowledge with gratitude the many people who have contributed their histories and experiences of bullying. Their bravery is outstanding. My good colleagues Iain Coyne and Elizabeth Seigne of the University of Hull have provided a significant body of research in relation to personality structure. Their efforts have opened up avenues of enquiry which will do much to extend our understanding of adult bullying.

I am grateful also to Professor Joel Newman of the State University of New York who gave me permission to use the model of workplace aggression which he evolved with Professor Robert Baron of the Rensselaer Polytechnic Institute. My thanks go also to Pat Lindley and Ken Danderfer of Prevue for permission to use material from the ICES manual.

My dear wife, Marilyn, deserves particular mention for her limitless help with preparation of the manuscript and insightful comments. Finally, I must thank my 12-year-old son, Graham, whose robust statements reassure me that the next generation is no more likely to tolerate bullying than mine.

P. E. Randall
November 2000

Introduction

This book largely concerns the well-researched area of workplace bullying and is divided into four parts. The first part is concerned with the problem of operational definitions and attempts to bring them together to enable the derivation of a model of adult bullying that enables a robust structure to guide assessment. The second and third parts examine the developmental and interpersonal experiences that are associated with the shaping of bully/victim traits and which may be unleashed by environmental contingencies. The final part deals with the clinical consequences of severe adult bullying and endeavours to unite settings, antecedents, behaviour and consequences through examples of assessment outcome. Inevitably such a structuring is forced and does not properly reflect the complexities of adult bullying but it has facilitated my own work with bullies and their victims.

Part I Definitions and assessment structure

Chapter I An overview of adult bullying

This chapter begins by attempting to draw together important operational definitions from around the world where workplace bullying is studied. Particular Scandinavian, Canadian, American and British inputs were chosen as representative but I acknowledge that these are not an exhaustive list. It is clear, however, that different conceptualisations and research formats yield similar results, and by linking them it becomes easier to study the significant variables that are associated with bully/victim problems and to present an overview that guides assessment procedures.

The first chapter summarises these variables and introduces also the consequences to both bullies and victims of this form of human aggression. There is a brief description of the legal context of this behaviour at the end of the first chapter; this is not intended to be a guide to the law but an indication of how there is now a powerful movement in litigation throughout the industrialised world which not only demands accurate assessments of individuals involved but constitutes also sets of antecedents (policy and practice requirements designed to inhibit workplace aggression) and powerful consequences in terms of potential court action.

Chapter 2 Workplace bullying as a variety of human aggression

This chapter makes use of the model of workplace aggression evolved by Joel Neuman and Robert Baron to provide a means of evolving a further model which enables bully/victim problems to be analysed according to settings, setting conditions, other important antecedents and reinforcing consequences. In so doing it is possible to propose that adult bullying in the workplace should not be studied as a unique phenomenon but as a variety of human aggression which has much in common with other forms.

Chapter 3 A framework for assessment

This chapter commences with a rationale for assessment which is based upon a fairly standard approach to the clinical investigation of psychological difficulties.

Into this is woven the issues that are of particular relevance to adult bullying. For the sake of clarity the model assumes that the environment for the alleged bullying is the workplace. Thus the assessment must include detail about the employment culture, stressing the organisational context of the bullying; the level of perceived task complexity and the awareness of line managers of the victim's experiences and their responses.

Details of the alleged incidents need to be given and analysed for their type and severity with reference to the detailed research on these issues.

The impact upon the victim of the alleged bullying is examined, again in the context of what is known of likely effects, such as post-traumatic symptoms and/or social anxiety disorder.

Psychometric assessment devices are introduced although details of their particular contribution are given in relevant later chapters.

This chapter then examines the derivation of the formulation from which conclusions follow.

Part 2 Characteristics of perpetrators

Chapter 4 Bully characteristics: personal history and development

This chapter covers the main 'ingredients' of life experience which contribute to the development of persistent interpersonal aggression which characterises the activity of adult bullies.

These include the bully's own experiences of being parented and the chapter examines the role of dysfunctional attachment as a primary antecedent to the development of the bullying personality type. Early temperamental characteristics are not forgotten in this chapter but weight is placed upon experiential factors in relation to the style of parenting received, particularly in respect of the early reinforcement of aggressive traits.

The consideration of personal history passes on to a consideration of the bully's own experiences, if any, of being bullied outside of the family and their prior history of bullying others. Attention is paid to reinforcing circumstances which are liable to heighten a predisposition to bullying which may arise from factors within the organisational culture of the workplace.

Chapter 5 Bully characteristics: personality traits

This chapter is concerned predominantly with attitudinal characteristics, and a model of assessing aggressive traits is reviewed. The relationship of bullying to personality disorders is investigated and comment is made upon the assessment of these. Antisocial and narcissistic personality disorders are described in the context of case studies relating these to workplace bullying.

A discussion of Theory of Mind factors follows which enables an assessment of those bullies who fail to realise the significance of their actions in relation to the psychological harm they cause. This is linked to organisational factors that can 'trigger' workplace aggression.

This chapter considers the use of the psychometric evaluation of some characteristics of a 'bully profile'.

Part 3 Characteristics of victims

Chapter 6 Victim characteristics: personal history and development

The chapter commences with a review of the victim's experiences of being parented and what this may mean in terms of dysfunctional attachments. An examination of the style of parenting received is important because of the evidence that associates this to a later history of being bullied.

The victim's history of being bullied as a child is considered, as is any history of being bullied in other contexts (e.g. other places of work, home, community). Factors relating to racial background, physical and sensory disabilities, intellectual/educational limitations and sexual orientation are considered in relation to the assessment process.

Chapter 7 Victim characteristics: personality factors

This chapter reviews the relevance of submissive and provocative victim personality types and relates these to the allegations of bullying, peer support (or the lack of it) and the opinions of line managers.

The assessment model requires also an investigation of the victim's characteristic responses to being bullied and examines these for trends which encourage the bullies.

A considerable part of this chapter examines the 'Victim Scale' derived from research studies with a particular personality inventory that is for use in employment environments. The use of this in formulating hypotheses for intervention is considered.

Part 4 Assessment outcomes and clinical consequences

Chapter 8 The effects of adult bullying

This chapter reviews the growing detail available of the effects of bullying and relates this to the assessment of damage in relation to psychological harm (e.g. PTSD, Social Anxiety Disorder); impact on employment prospects and continuation of a career; the effects on observers of witnessing repeated workplace bullying; and the impact on family members of victims.

Chapter 9 The report: assessment outcomes

This chapter presents the collation of assessment findings through an intermediate report. This is supported by two detailed case reports which are accompanied by relevant commentary.

Part 1

Definitions and assessment structure

Chapter 1

An overview of adult bullying

One of the most startling impressions of even a cursory scan of case files concerning adult bullying is the ingenuity that perpetrators have shown in finding ways of inflicting misery on their victims. There appears to be an almost boundless set of strategies for causing harm and an infinite supply of enthusiasm available for doing so. Although many adult bullies are simple opportunists, there are as many whose Machiavellian talents are put to use in finding devious ways of bringing pain to their victims without discredit to themselves.

Almost as startling, the scan of cases reveals a frightening creativity amongst the reasons victims are given for what happens to them. The workplace bully of today need not be the brutish, ignorant thug that the stereotype of yesterday would have us believe. Although some are, and use physical intimidation instead of negotiation, many workplace bullies can be subtle, charming, intelligent and even sensitive. They can accurately predict the feelings of others; they can understand the pain they cause but they just do not care. Their understanding is used to better hone their weapons and their portrayal of empathy is just a means of preserving their own credibility.

Perhaps because victims feel easier these days about 'coming out', the number involved has also become deeply worrying. Incidence figures appear to be rising but may actually only reflect this greater willingness to admit to victim status. Even so, it is a frightening commentary on workplace environments that some findings indicate bullying to be one of the largest single causes of absenteeism.

Increasingly research and clinical experience demonstrate that the tide of human misery caused by bullying is not just felt by the direct victims. Others suffer as well; close family members, for example, watch a saddening change steal over their mothers, fathers and partners; they witness a slow decline from the victim's normal presentation through anger to anxiety and then depression. They watch humour and confidence ebb away to be replaced by low mood and fearfulness. The quality of their relationships suffer as the victims lose their sense of self and become more introspective, continually asking 'Why me? What's wrong with me?' Children gradually lose their parent playmates and partners their best friends.

Within the workplace, passive observers suffer also; those who do not collude with the bullies wonder if or when it will be their turn as their workplace environment deteriorates around them. For many of these passive observers, painful memories of their own experiences of being bullied, or being bullies, surface as unwelcome memories that had been deeply buried. They recall times at school or college when they were victims or perpetrators, revisit events of the past, which they had learned from, then left behind.

Every incident of bullying is like a stone dropped in a pool. The immediate impact is the harm done to the direct victim; the ripples represent the disturbance around the victim–bully dyad, widening out to the damage done to others and ultimately, where senior management remains passive or colludes, to the whole culture of the organisation.

This book is concerned with adult bullying and the assessments of those who experience it as victims and those who inflict it. Adults are anyone who is 18 years or more old and at work. For a variety of reasons 'work' also includes educational environments where the people involved may be students or staff. In the main, workplace bullying is focused upon as it is a particularly well-researched field of enquiry and attracts the attention of human services practitioners as well as academics. Bullying is not a unique phenomenon; it is an example of a wide range of behaviour loosely labelled 'human aggression'. This theme is described in Chapter 2, whilst this chapter seeks only to provide an overview of workplace bullying, its antecedents and consequences.

Operational definitions

The word 'bullying' defies a completely satisfactory definition because it has been used in many different ways over generations of English language users. Often used as synonymous with 'harassment', the verb 'to harass' itself is no less confused. To harass is thought to be related to the old French verb 'harer', meaning 'to set a dog on', and it has links also with the Old English word 'hergian', meaning to ravage and despoil. Indeed, 'Old Harry' is an archaic synonym for the Devil which is derived also from 'hergian'. In more recent English usage, a bully is defined as habitually cruel or overbearing, especially to smaller or weaker people. A bully may also have been a pimp or a hired thug. It is strange that these relatively modern meanings should have been preceded by others such as 'a fine person' or a 'sweetheart'. To Shakespeare, a bully was a brisk, jovial and dashing person.

Scientific formalisation has lent little resolution to the problem of definition. As has been pointed out on many occasions (e.g. Rayner, Sheehan and Barker, 1999), there is no agreed definition of bullying. In part this is due to the different stances taken by researchers who, in focusing on their own particular area, develop definitions that fit best. Thus, clinical studies have led to one operational definition (e.g. Randall, 1997) and studies of severe trauma in bullying have led to another (e.g. Zapf, Knorz and Kulla, 1996). Rayner (1997) examined bullying from the primary investigation viewpoint of its incidence, whilst other researchers concern themselves with environmental antecedents as initiators of a spectrum of human aggressive behaviours (e.g. Baron and Neuman, 1996). In addition, Liefooghe and Olafsson (1999, 1.1) examined the views of non-bullied personnel and concluded that the behaviour labelled 'bullying' may vary from one organisation to another. Mehta (2000) using a novel application of grounded theory, found evidence that what is conceptualised as bullying may vary from individual to individual working within the same department of an employing organisation.

Even within these areas of application, the term 'bullying' may become further differentiated. Thus Einarsen (2000) distinguished between predatory and dispute-related bullying. Predatory bullying is often the simple abuse of power of a stronger individual over a vulnerable person who apparently has done nothing to justify the aggression. Victims are targeted because they can be bullied with little cost to the bullies. Dispute-related bullying, however, arises out of real or imagined grievances and is initiated by conflicts within the workplace. As will be seen, however, clinical studies further confuse this simple dichotomy by showing how the boundaries between dispute-related and predatory bullying blur depending on the differing perspectives of victims and bullies. There is little doubt, however, that, whatever definitions may be used, bullying is an aggressive behaviour which is characterised in general by repetition and an imbalance of power (e.g. Smith and Brain, 2000).

Not surprisingly definitions vary also according to predominant schools of thought and experimental design. These have become identifiable almost on a country by country basis. Four of these are considered here.

The first was provided by the author in a previous book (Randall, 1997a) as '*Bullying is the aggressive behaviour arising from the deliberate intent to cause physical or psychological distress to others.*' This definition deals with motivational factors and describes the purpose behind the bully's intentional actions. The following case is an example.

Lynn was a 48-year-old section supervisor for a metropolitan authority. She was brought before a disciplinary committee on two occasions for alleged breaches of the Personal Harassment policy. On both occasions there was insufficient evidence to take action. Most people would have taken heed of these events as a warning but Lynn did not. The third complaint against her was substantiated. Although she kept her job she was required to speak to an independent counsellor. Finally she was able to admit: 'I was sick of the youngsters coming in with their degrees and happy faces. They knew nothing at all about showing proper respect to someone like me, an older person who had worked up from clerical assistant grade. They needed a bit of pushing around to wipe the smug smiles off their faces and understand how life really is. I was doing them a favour and I didn't mind being cruel to be kind. Yes, I gave them as much menial work as I could – why not? They got good at it; that's something to be proud of, isn't it? But they say I threatened them – what sort of a world is it where a manager can't use a few threats to get things done. OK, so I made them cancel holidays and criticised them for staying at home when their kids were sick. They shouldn't have kids and a job; one or the other will suffer and I don't see why it should be my section. A bit of pain did them good – they'll thank me for it one day'.

Clearly this individual has the intention to cause harm, arising from purely personal motivation, and the opportunity to do so. Cognitive dissonance, the bully's best friend, operates to help her feel that she is providing a valuable life lesson, a favour.

The second definition is descriptive of a variety of behaviour and does not require any consideration of internal mediation events such as motivation and intentionality. The Scandinavian tradition for both school-based and workplace bullying is to consider 'mobbing' or group bullying. The main factors of this are present in the process definition given by Leymann as *'social interaction through which one person (seldom more) is attacked by one or more (seldom more than four) individuals almost on a daily basis and for periods of many months, bringing the person into an almost helpless position with potentially high risk of expulsion'* (Leymann, 1996, p. 168). Leymann argues that mobbing is a psychological 'terror' brought to victims through 'hostile and unethical communication, which is directed in a systematic way by one or a few individuals' (p. 168). The victims are forced into a defenceless position in which they are held by the mobbing strategies adopted. Psychological harm is likely to be sustained by these victims who may experience psychosomatic symptoms as well as social negation. Leymann points out that the essence of mobbing as a destroyer of human beings lies not so much in what is done but in the frequency and duration of what is done. It may be seen, therefore, that seemingly mild verbal harassment can become psychologically damaging if used systematically by a group on a frequent basis over a long period of time.

The following gives a case work example:

'I know Rob took it to Personnel and was saying we bullied him. They didn't do much about it anyway – in fact he was offered a transfer which he didn't take, the silly sod. Yes, I know we ragged him for months but that's nothing, is it?

We do a rough job; it's rugged being out all day in all weathers. The public have no idea what it's like keeping the roads moving. They just stay in their warm cars and watch the lovely country passing by – they don't have a clue how cold, wet and thoroughly bloody miserable it is a lot of the time. We have to be tough.

Puffs don't fit in our gang – we are a crude lot; none of us is going to win a charm award. What the hell did he expect once the lads found out he was gay. Can't he take a joke without going all soppy with his nerves. I blame management.'

This last example deals with a foreman of a road repair and maintenance crew. He had little time for anyone who did not fit within his constructs of manliness and so a gay man, Robert, was an ideal target for him. His crew members were only too pleased to join in and 'mobbing' resulted. Their homophobic insults, or 'jokes' as they described them, were made all the more threatening by frequent shoves and excessively hard back-slapping.

Robert was subjected to a lengthy process of vilification which led ultimately to exclusion.

The third definition comes from a parallel and equally valid contribution from Canada. Keashly (1998) aligns most of the behaviours listed by European researchers as workplace bullying or mobbing under the label of *emotional abuse*. This term was chosen because it appears to reflect the severe and long-term consequences to victims that are evident in their narrations and because it is readily differentiated from physical, sexual and racial abuse which are delineated by the 'form and context of the behaviours used against people' (Keashly, 1998, p. 88). Keashly notes the importance of the fact that many of these emotionally abusive behaviours in the workplace are often group behaviours with descriptions not unlike those included under workplace bullying and mobbing. In differentiating the emotionally abusive behaviours of the workplace from the serious criminal behaviours of physical, sexual and racial abuse, Keashly is referring to similar behaviours which have occupied European researchers. Her summary table (Keashly, 1998, pp. 97–98) provides an excellent sample of studies of international origin, reflecting the diversity of bullying behaviours that may be considered 'emotional abuse'.

Keashly provides seven dimensions or elements of definitions that appear to be incorporated within studies of non-physical abuse in the workplace. She argues that these elements of definition give rise to testable hypotheses about the construct of emotional abuse.

On examination, these seem to be perfectly valid for those defining characteristics of other labels of workplace harassment used elsewhere.

1   **'Emotional abuse includes verbal and nonverbal modes of expression'**
    (Keashly, 1998, p. 96): Verbal forms include direct forms such as yelling
    and screaming at targeted people as well as the use of insults, tantrums
    and rudeness. More subtle forms include accusations of wrongdoing,
    blaming for errors and belittling. Indirect forms include rumour-
    mongering, gossip, breaching confidentiality, withholding necessary
    information and taking credit for work tasks.

    Non-verbal forms include glaring, ignoring (silent treatment), intimi-
    datory physical gestures (such as finger pointing, slamming objects down
    on surfaces) and throwing objects.

    Keashly lists studies associated with these forms and pays particular
    heed to the work of Baron and Neuman (1996) who make use of the
    framework for categorising human aggression developed by Buss (1961).
    This important work is described in Chapter 2.

    Keashly describes the outcomes of an unpublished study which indi-
    cates that verbal direct forms of aggression (such as yelling, screaming
    and insulting) are viewed by employees as being more abusive than forms
    such as glaring or ignoring.

2   **'Behaviours are emotionally abusive when they are of a repeated nature**
    or part of a pattern' (Keashly, 1998, p. 101): Keashly's own research
    experience of this dimension accords well with other research employing
    narrative data (e.g. Randall, 1997a). Her experience is congruent with the
    perception of victims that even comparatively mild behaviours become
    abusive if they are encountered on a frequent (e.g. daily) basis. The more
    severe the behaviour the less frequently it has to occur before being
    branded as abusive. Randall (1997) gives as an example the plight of a
    prisoner being threatened with his life only once by a vicious inmate as
    being exceptionally intimidatory.

    Clearly, the repeated nature of behaviours being perceived as aggres-
    sive fits well with the conceptualisation of mobbing as provided by
    Leymann (1996).

3   **'Behaviours are emotionally abusive when they are unwelcome and**
    unsolicited' (Keashly, 1998, p. 103): Keashly points out that none of
    the behaviours listed could be viewed as desirable or wanted. Yet, it is the
    case that most personal harassment policies of employers require that the
    victim make a clear statement that they are unwanted. The legal context
    of bullying is explored later in this chapter but the important psycho-
    logical issue is whether or not the victim has acted in a particular way to
    encourage the harassment. Although this seems trite, the author has come
    across bully–victim dyads who act in concert to meet each other's needs –
    a situation that is better examined using social exchange theory (e.g.
    Frude, 1992; Lawler and Thye, 1999) than a theory of human aggression.

    A major issue in this area of investigation concerns the elicitation of
    anger and the narratives of victims and bullies can provide very different

perspectives on this. As Keashly points out, it is invariably the case that the respective narratives of bully and victim are shaped to minimise their respective responsibility for the harassment behaviour. In the author's experience, for example, irritated line managers defend their constant rebuking of poorly performing individuals as part of their role, whereas those individuals perceive this as unwelcome harassment.

4   'Behaviours are emotionally abusive when they violate a standard of appropriate contact towards others' (Keashly, 1998, p. 104): International research into workplace bullying supports this dimension from all strategies of research endeavour. Some behaviours are perceived to be completely inappropriate in all workplaces although others may be perceived differently across different types of workplaces. Thus being made to stand to attention when being given instructions could be unacceptable in a local authority social services office but would be regarded as acceptable in the Armed Forces. Conversely, being insulted or having one's personal life exposed to public scrutiny are types of harassment that are viewed as unacceptable across all employment situations.

5   'Behaviours are emotionally abusive when they result in harm or injury to the target' (Keashly, 1998, p. 106): There is international research support for this dimension in relation to workers' opinions about immediate harm or injury. Not so obvious, but none the less important, is the psychological harm done by repeated harassment of a non-physical variety. There is extensive evidence that a variety of post-traumatic stress can result from frequent harassment (e.g. Randall, 1997) and this is evident throughout studies of harassment irrespective of what label is used for the aggression. The legal connotations of this are obvious although complex; people will endeavour to sue if they believe that they have experienced serious provable harm of any sort as a consequence of harassment. The complexity arises out of the need to demonstrate that the physical and/or psychological harm was the result of the harassment or due wholly or in part to other causes or pre-existing conditions.

Despite these difficulties, however, it is the case that research throughout the industrialised world shows that aggressive behaviours at work which cause such harm are indicative of abuse whether or not it is called emotional abuse, mobbing or workplace bullying.

6   'Behaviours are emotionally abusive when the aggressor intended to harm the target or allowed harmful events to be experienced by the target' (Keashly, 1998, p. 108): Keashly considers here the issue of intention and states that the more victims believe their harassment to have been intended to cause or allow them to experience harm, the more they are likely to perceive abuse. This resonates well with narrative studies of adult bullying which give rise to definitions that incorporate intention (e.g. Randall, 1997).

7   'Behaviours are emotionally abusive when the bully is in a more powerful

position relative to the victim' (Keashly, 1998, p. 109): Keashly acknow-
ledges that power is not always that of organisational or position power.
Although harassment is most frequently perpetrated by line managers
against their staff, position power is not the only power type. Other forms
of power may be influential, including 'referent power', that granted to
individuals by others who perceive some traits as being particularly
effective. For example, Raven (1992) suggests that some individuals exert
power that is not derived from their formal position in the organisation.
They are given this power by others who perceive them to have some
qualities which set them apart from the norm. These qualities can be
positive (e.g. effective leadership) or negative (e.g. domineering, aggressive). Their actions may determine unofficial working practices and set
the general climate of the department or organisation. Once again, this
dimension and the research support for it accord well with the narratives
of bullies and victims (e..g., Randall, 1997) and also provide a further
dimension to the role of intention (i.e. the intent to cause harm by the
deliberate misuse of power).

This valuable exercise of theoretical dissection creates important avenues
for further research which Keashly identifies as necessary in order to establish
antecedent links (e.g. do violations of standards lead to harm?) which
would provide credibility to the construct of workplace aggression as well
as emotional abuse. Although narrative studies are highly supportive of
her definitional elements, appropriate empirical work is the *sine qua non* of
scientific progress and this remains to be completed. In the meantime it is
sufficient to retain the construct as a possible source of operational guidance
and hence as a viable description of workplace bullying.

Workplace aggression

The fourth definitional consideration comes from the work of Robert Baron
and Joel Neuman which provides an American input of great importance to
the deliberations on workplace bullying. Their conceptualisations are closer
to those of the author than others but from different empirical formulations.
Their theme, that workplace aggression is not unique but a subset of
behaviours within the generic domain of human aggression, is distilled from
empirical studies, whereas the similar theme of the author is derived from
clinical observation and narrative.

The work of Baron and Neuman is considered in detail in Chapter 2 but
the item of particular importance to this section is their definition of workplace aggression. Given their theme concerning human aggression in general,
they accept that this involves any act in which an individual *intentionally*
attempts to harm another (Neuman and Baron, 1998). The key element of
intentionality immediately opens up a unifying pathway to the operational

definition of the present author (as given above). Their own operational definition states that *workplace aggression* is defined as *'efforts by individuals to harm others with whom they work, or have worked, or the organisations in which they are presently, or were previously, employed'* (Neuman and Baron, 1998, p. 395).

Unification of operational definitions

The fact that four major considerations of bullying in the workplace can lead to operational definitions or categorisations which share a close literature and research base is indicative of the degree to which international opinion is shared. It is indicative also of the degree to which different research investigations yield similar findings.

The operational definition which has guided the author's work is the first provided above; this choice is not based on a belief that it is better but simply on familiarity; in practice any of the definitions would suffice to assist the development of an affective model to guide the investigation of the dysfunctional set of adult interpersonal relationships that this author chooses to refer to as 'workplace bullying'.

The nature of bullying behaviour

Within the definition of bullying, the variety of bullying behaviour seems endless. It is helpful at the institutional level to categorise them. On the basis of large-scale survey work, the TUC (1998) put forward three categories to facilitate descriptions of bullying behaviour. These fit well with the operational definition given above. Bullying:

- undermines professional ability (work skills) in front of other staff;
- creates extra work or otherwise disrupts the victim's ability to work;
- isolates staff.

As will be seen, the majority of case work examples given throughout this book can be summarised by one or more of these categories of bullying behaviour.

There are dangers, however, in making an assumption that specific examples of bullying will always fit within these three categories. It would not be wise to exclude any behaviours that did not fit within them as being something other than bullying. There is evidence that forms of perceived bullying differ from one organisational context to another (Liefooghe and Olafsson, 1999) and it is also the case that lay people do not share the same appreciation of which behaviours count as 'bullying' amongst the adult working population. It is these people, of course, who interpret the behaviours they witness or experience directly as bullying or some form of negative events, and bring them to the attention of their employers. Naturally enough, they do not work to operational definitions as they do so, and victims particularly will be less able to use objectivity in considering what has happened to them. Thus not only is there a variation about perceived bullying behaviour within the organisation context but also between individuals.

Einarsen (1999) reports on research which suggests five categories of bullying behaviour:

1   work-related bullying which may include changing the victim's work tasks or making them harder;
2   social isolation;
3   personal attacks and attacks on the victim's private life, ridicule, gossip, insulting comments, etc.;
4   verbal assaults such as public criticism, yelling and similar humiliations;
5   physical assaults or threats of physical harm.

The resemblance to the definitional elements of Keashly is clear. This categorisation means little to traumatised victims whose experiences have overwhelmed them. Many would not recognise the sophisticated manipulation of others in any of these, leading not to social isolation but to inclusion within a group of other victims accepted within an underclass stretching from shop floor to management hierarchy.

In addition, victims point out that many of the behaviours of bullying are only a little removed from everyday living experiences; being criticised at work or yelled at by an angry person is something that most people experience from time to time. It may be distressing at the time but does not result in trauma or victim status. As described, Leymann (1996) and Randall (1997a) have pointed out that bullying behaviours may not be abnormal in type but that the severity and/or frequency makes them damaging. To complicate the matter further, case work studies reveal that severity need not relate to the intensity of the behaviours directed against the victim but the status of the . person using it. It is no accident that many surveys reveal that bullies are more commonly to be found amongst the managers of victims. One study was carried out in an NHS Community Trust in the UK and was comprised of a questionnaire survey made up of an inventory of bullying behaviours specifically designed for the study; a work-induced scale for stress; an anxiety and depression scale; a job satisfaction scale; and other measures examining degree of support at work and propensity to leave the job. These were returned by 1,100 employees which was a very substantial response rate of 70 per cent. Thirty-eight per cent of employees had experiences of one or more types of bullying and 42 per cent had witnessed them. The bullying was most likely to be carried out by a senior manager or line manager and it was the antecedent of lower levels of job satisfaction and higher levels of job-induced stress, depression and desire to leave the job (Quine, 1999).

This finding concerning management bullying is supported by practice-led enquiry and, with specific reference again to the NHS, Lockhart (1997) describes the work of a Staff Support Service and provides three clear case studies of bullying by management staff.

The bulk of workplace bullying incidents shows the bully as a manager and the victim as a subordinate (Einarsen, 1999) and evidence exists that victims suffer more from this than from the bullying of co-workers (e.g. Einarsen and Raknes, 1997). Both empirical and case study investigations demonstrate that the severity of bullying behaviour is related also to characteristics or circumstances of the victim. Research suggests that personal factors such as economics or physical circumstances may operate to make victims more vulnerable and less able to defend themselves. Victims' perception of the severity of being bullied is influenced also by their own history of being bullied (e.g. Einarsen and Skogstad, 1996; Randall, 1997) and their previous recovery from it (Randall and Parker, 2000). Where that recovery is poor and the history of bullying remains alive in the victim's mind, then further incidents have an enhanced negative effect.

It is clear that the factors that influence victims' perceptions of bullying behaviour are complex and interactive. There is a view that the complexities are such that 'bullying' is not open to explanation on the basis of a single set of theoretical concepts, nor can it be defined in a manner that fulfils scientific criteria. Case study narratives, however, give painful evidence that victims fully understand their tormentors' intentions to cause them harm and the processes by which they do so.

The incidence of workplace bullying

Counsellors of the victims of workplace bullying assert that it helps their clients to know that there are others who experience similar assaults on their dignity, self-esteem and life opportunities. It is generally agreed that the incidence of workplace bullying is far greater than was ever thought. The Scandinavian research teams are probably the longest involved in this area; Einarsen and Skogstad (1996), for example, examined fourteen different surveys in Norway and found that 8.6 per cent of respondents had been subjected to workplace bullying within the previous six months. Vartia (1996) carried out a survey in Finland and reported a rate of 10.1 per cent. Rayner (1997) carried out a survey of 1,137 respondents at a university in the UK in 1994; nearly half of the sample reported that they had been bullied at some point in their working lives and many reported being bullied in groups, a finding which runs contrary to narrative evidence.

Some writers (e.g. Field, 1997) claim that bullying in the UK has reached epidemic proportions. Evidence is drawn from the results of the TUC hotline concerning 'Bad Bosses'. This is said to have logged 5,000 calls in five days from all walks of working life. Of these, 38 per cent were about bullying. As support for a higher frequency rate in the UK, the results of a study by Edelmann and Woodall (1997) of the 172 members of the Professional Association of Teachers found a high rate of 18.7 per cent. The outcomes of Quine's study of 1999 are even more distressing. As reported previously, Quine carried out a large survey of the employees of an NHS Community Trust and had a response rate of 70 per cent to the questionnaires sent out. Of these, 38 per cent reported experiencing one or more types of bullying during the course of the previous year. In addition, 42 per cent had witnessed others being bullied. Examination of the characteristics of the victims reveals that no occupational group escaped; thus, although 31 per cent of the doctors were or had been bullied, as opposed to 44 per cent of nurses, they still experienced being bullied. It would appear that level or occupational status is no protection for individuals.

None of these figures should be treated as more accurate than the others. The lack of agreed operational definition bedevils cross-study comparison. For example, whilst there is general agreement that there should be repetitive aversive behaviour (e.g. Einarsen and Skogstad, 1996; Leymann, 1996) there is little agreement on the duration of persistence. Leymann (1992) requires a minimum of six months, whilst Bjorkqvist, Osterman and Hjelt-Bäck (1994) set their criteria as one year. Einarsen and Skogstad (1996) require only that the aversive behaviour has occurred at some point over a six-month period.

In respect of school-based bullying, many researchers (e.g. Randall, 1996; Smith and Sharp, 1994) follow the criteria set by Olweus (1989) for his national survey across Norway. Issues of frequency are also problematic, with tight criteria being set by some researchers, such as Leymann (1996) who requires a weekly incidence, whereas others are much looser. Randall (1997), for example, argued that severity of low-frequency bullying can be very damaging and more important than frequency.

The effects of workplace bullying on victims

There is an increasing body of research and clinical narrative evidence which indicates the serious effects of workplace bullying on individuals. Niedl (1996) found from a sample of 368 Austrian hospital employees that victims showed significantly greater evidence of reduced well-being than non-victims. Their symptoms included anxiety, irritation, depression and psychosomatic complaints. This finding was repeated in a German study (Zapf, Knorz and Kulla, 1996). Einarsen and Raknes (1997) reported a negative association for male shipyard workers between exposure to victimisation at work and psychological health and well-being.

The UK study of teachers by Edelmann and Woodall (1997) provided a more detailed picture of effects: 44.2 per cent of the sample reported loss of confidence, 38 per cent reported more physical ailments whilst 37.2 per cent experienced stress. Long-term psychological and/or physical effects were found in 53.5 per cent whilst 21.5 per cent developed an inability to cope. Lowered self-esteem was experienced by 19.8 per cent of the sample – a surprisingly low proportion in contrast with clinical narrative evidence which suggests that virtually all long-term victims of workplace bullying had low self-confidence or developed it. Clinical studies reveal that loss of self-esteem is a frequent and devastating product of the bullying and can happen to the strongest of people, as this example demonstrates.

'I was a serving officer in a very active regiment for fifteen years. I saw action in Northern Ireland, the Falklands and the Gulf as well as a few other places the public never heard of. By the age of 45 and in Civvy street I honestly didn't believe that any aggressive people could get the better of me.

I couldn't have been more wrong when I started [at a security firm] and began working for a woman general manager. I'm not saying all woman managers were like her but she was evil incarnate.

She lost no opportunity to slag off my work, overrule my decisions and patronise me. My leave was cancelled with twenty-four hours' notice and I wasn't allowed time off to go to my son's sports day. She always had excuses and reminded me charmingly that this was business and not the military with a guaranteed budget. When I complained about her antics she went and cried in the office of her boss. I got into hot water with him and it wasn't until one of the changed decisions lost a big contract that he got wise to her. By that time I felt totally useless and as green as a raw recruit. I lost confidence and feared to take any decisions.'

Psychological and physical ill-health are frequent consequences of any form of prolonged stress. The experience of being bullied is no exception. The recent TUC study (1998) reports on headaches, anxiety, raised blood pressure, nausea, sleep disorder and suicidal ideation. Some researchers (e.g. Leymann and Gustafsson, 1996; Randall, 1997) comment on symptoms that fit within the diagnostic criteria (DSM-IV) of Post-Traumatic Stress Disorder (PTSD). These include cognitive dysfunction, mainly of memory and attention control; stress effects including sweating and chest pains; psychosomatic effects including headaches, neck-aches and stiffness as well as sleep disorder; avoidance reactions and emotional lability. These effects may permeate all aspects of the victim's life, not just the workplace.

The effects on individuals of harassment have been well recorded over many years. For example, Brodsky (1976) recorded three types of effects on victims. Some experienced indeterminate physical symptoms including loss of strength, chronic tiredness, aches and pains and other difficulties. Others experienced depression and depression-related difficulties such as loss of self-esteem, sleep disorder and impotence. The third group experienced hyperactivity, feelings of hostility, a wish to avoid social contacts, anxiety and feelings of victimisation. There were considerable individual differences which suggest that personality factors operate as moderators.

The effect on individuals, whether they are direct victims or witness others being bullied, can be severe. Estimates suggest that bullying accounts for between one-third and a half of stress-related sickness absence. It appears to be associated with lowered productivity rates, poor staff morale and an increase in staff turnover. Many writers have pointed out that competitive organisations can ill afford such effects and stress the need for properly policed anti-bullying policies (e.g. Randall, 1997).

The antecedents of workplace bullying

Personality factors

Much of the research into the reasons why this behaviour should occur has examined organisational factors. Leymann (1996) is opposed to the possibility that personality factors related to the victims could be antecedents and suggests that abnormalities of personality may arise because of the bullying rather than being an antecedent of it. Vartia (1996) disagrees and states that there is a need to study the possible role of personality variables and suggests that these may be of particular importance when victims are 'selected'. Case work evidence shows that personality factors can be influential; many victims in the writer's experience are able to define precisely why they were selected because the bullies have told them. These samples of clinical narrative are illustrative of this point.

'The main bully was the charge hand; he told me straight that he didn't like people who get upset easily and worry a lot. He said his section was better off without them.'

'She said it was fun to get at people like me who were quiet and didn't say much.'

'I like to work all the time; it stops me getting bored. They said they would drive me out because I made them look slow.'

In support of influential personality factors, Vartia (1996) reported a negative correlation between bullying and Neuroticism with victims showing higher N scores than a non-bullied sample. This correlation was reduced when work environment and climate were controlled but remained to a degree. Brodsky (1976) believed that people bullied at work were more likely to be conscientious, literal-minded, paranoid, rigid and compulsive. Similarly Coyne, Seigne and Randall (2000a) showed that victims tended to be less independent and extroverted and more unstable and more conscientious than non-victims. This work is vital to the assessment of victims and will be discussed in more detail in a later chapter. Certainly there is significant support for a personality influence from studies of school-based bullying. For example, Slee and Rigby (1993) gave eighty-seven Australian male primary school children the Junior Personality Inventory. Victims scored significantly below both 'normal' children and bullies on Extroversion whereas bullies scored more highly on the Psychoticism scale. The latter is highly associated with anti-social interactions and lowered empathy. Mynard and Joseph (1997) were able to replicate these findings in respect of Extroversion and noted that victims tended to have higher (not significant) scores on the Neuroticism scale. Byrne (1994), using a sample of children from schools in Dublin, reported that victims were more withdrawn and more neurotic than both bullies and controls. Olafsen and Viemero (2000) found that coping strategies of aggression and self-destruction typified bullies and victims.

Personality tests have been used to test for personality differences; for example, Gandolfo (1995) compared MMPI-2 profiles of American victims of harassment who were claiming compensation with the profiles of other complainants who had not been harassed. The harassed complainants were more suspicious, over-sensitive and angry than the controls. Both groups, however, showed evidence of depression and psychosomatic symptoms.

Organisational factors

These can be sufficient conditions for workplace bullying. Vartia (1996), for example, reports that the strains of highly competitive environments tend to be associated with workplace bullying. This is borne out by evidence of case studies as these comments from victims indicate:

'The work is set up in such a way that you have to grab for parts to slot in the circuits as they come down the line. The bullies just take what they want off the other workers. Anyone who complains is threatened with violence.'

'The sales manager sets out to pit us one against the other; he encourages us to be aggressive and talks about weeding the softies out.'

'I used to like playing football for the works; not now. The coach goes

> on and on about winning; he screams at anyone who drops below his standards and pushes and shoves them.'
>
> 'I came into this job to help people. The senior social worker says this is crap – we are here to get things done for next to nothing and I'd better not rock his boat.'

Brodsky's view from the 1970s is as apposite now. Her view was that harassment was an institutional phenomenon which regarded harassment as a legitimate means of securing compliance. In addition, she viewed this behaviour as a means of maintaining status within organisations

> If the pecking order indicates that those above shall have the right to annoy or displace those below, and if there is no pecking order and no harassment, then one must find other symbols of status. The privilege to harass is an inexpensive way of conferring status requiring no capital investment or outlay .... Because of this, harassment has become part of most management systems.
>
> (Brodsky, 1976, p. 7)

If this is true then it is not surprising that management styles have a lot of influence on bullying rates. For example, where management leads to role conflict alone with poor leadership and inadequate control of work loads then the resulting unpleasant climate can be associated with bullying (Einarsen, Raknes and Matthiesen, 1994). A hostile environment is associated also with insecurity in the workplace as, for example, when redundancies are threatened. This issue is discussed in Chapter 2.

Scandinavian research has tended to focus heavily on the importance of organisational factors and the social environment of the workplace. Einarsen (2000) reports that this situational perspective describes workplace bullying as caused by organisational and social problems. Leymann (1996) is a forceful advocate of this position and believes that personality factors are of little importance, victims being selected by force of circumstance only. Although this view does not find favour with all researchers it is a valid point that in the absence of longitudinal studies there is little evidence to suggest that abnormal personality variables cause victim selection or are simply the result of being bullied. Another possibility is that personality, social and organisational variables interact to define target selection.

Some large-scale studies implicating organisational and social variables have been carried out in Europe. For example, the study by Einarsen, Raknes and Matthiesen (1994) used over 2,000 subjects from six trade unions. Their analyses revealed that the recurrence of bullying was related to role conflict, leadership and social environment. Organisational factors of influence included ambiguity, incompatible demands and inappropriate expectations about rules and responsibilities, all of which create frustrations and conflicts. Not surprisingly bullies also expressed the same dissatisfactions in the author's own narrative studies, which begs the question as to why some people should become victims and others become bullies if the same antecedent variables are at work on both groups.

The Finnish study by Vartia (1996), mentioned above, provided findings comparable with the Einarsen study. Nearly 1,000 municipal employees provided results indicating that authoritarian dispute resolution, poor information transfer, lack of participation in discussion, and low influence in respect of work practices were all characteristics of employment environments in which bullying flourished. Similarly Zapf, Knorz and Kulla (1996) produced results from German victims which implicated a lack of control over their own time, being forced to work in an area of unresolved conflict and dissatisfaction with job content.

Previous beliefs about the role of routine, rushed and monotonous work associated with workplace conflicts (e.g. Appelberg, Romanov, Honlasalo and Koskenvuo, 1991) have been modified by more recent findings which indicate that it is the lack of opportunity to monitor and control work output that is frustrating when combined with poor leadership and similar variables. Neuman and Baron (1998) review these and other social/organisational variables (see also Chapter 2) including the influence of group norms that are permissive of hostility and conflict.

The legal context

This section is not designed to provide an authoritative text on the legislation as it relates to workplace bullying. Such a complex objective is best tackled by specialists in employment law. For example, Leighton (1999) provides an excellent description of the relevant legislation and there is little point in replication of such work here. This section, therefore, should not be taken as a definitive statement or interpretation of the law on bullying in general or in any particular case.

The legal context of workplace bullying cannot be ignored when assessments are made of bullies, victims and the environments in which the bullying takes place. The fact that legislation does exist to secure the rights of workplace victims is a potential antecedent to the vigorous efforts employers should make in respect of prevention. It is also a powerful provider of such consequences that victims everywhere can see justice being done.

More to the point of assessments, however, the legal context of workplace bullying provides guidance to the assessors of what information should be sought. Is the resulting psychological damage temporary or permanent? Do pre-existing mental health conditions muddy the clarity of individual cases? Do organisational factors predispose line managers and supervisors to

bullying behaviours? And have the victims made full use of whatever personnel support policies employers have put in place? These are major issues and
this is by no means an exhaustive list. Although psychologists should not
attempt to be lawyers and vice versa, it is often the case that each needs the
other to ensure that the strengths and weaknesses of workplace bullying cases
are fully investigated and expounded.

The writer has often found it odd that bullying has a clearer-cut place in
legislation relating to the protection of children and young people at school
than it does within the far broader domain of employment. In part this may
well be because bullying is often assumed to be a phenomenon of childhood
and not something that adults experience. Indeed there has been a particular
reluctance amongst Americans and Canadians to accept the term 'bullying'
because of the presumed connotations of school behaviour. Although this
view is changing, many employees, employers and professional support staff
prefer the term 'harassment'.

Despite the looser legal structure, a similar concept exists in educational
and employment legislation; this is the concept of a 'duty of care' owed to
students and employees alike. Teachers are *in loco parentis* which requires that
they exercise the same care as would a reasonable parent. Similarly, employers must endeavour to meet the welfare needs of their employees. It is
instructive to spend some time on a brief summary of the situation regarding
students at school.

Legislation and bullying at school

All teachers are taught during training about being *in loco parentis* and are
aware of their duty of care in respect of the physical and moral welfare of
pupils. The UK standard of care they are required to show is that of a careful
parent in respect of the avoidance of foreseeable damage and dangers. The
governors and headteachers of all schools have a duty of care to pupils to
enable them to study in safety. This duty of care includes the maintenance of
such measures as are necessary to prevent and/or ameliorate any indiscipline
that contravenes the behavioural standards of the school. Section 22 of the
Education (No. 2) Act, 1986 gives each headteacher the duty to encourage
good behaviour and respect for others[1] on the part of pupils. Bullying, which
is a variety of premeditated interpersonal aggression, is obviously a contra-
vention of such standards and prevents safe study within the school
environment.

There has been a significant volume of guidance material in UK schools to

---

1 The words 'and respect for others' were inserted by the Education Act 1993 (Schedule 19,
 para. 95).

facilitate the growing awareness of bullying amongst staff. All schools were sent a copy of *Good Behaviour and Discipline in Schools*, Education Observed No. 5 (DES), which deals in depth with the subject of indiscipline in the context of school ethos. In addition, *Attendance at School*, Education Observed No. 13 (DES) dealt with the issue of bullying as a factor associated with inattendance and made the point that parents have the right to expect teachers to take action on the problem if it is a cause of absenteeism.

Of greater significance than these documents, however, is the Elton Report (1989), *Discipline in Schools* (DES and Welsh Office, HMSO), which all schools were given. This deals with bullying in sections 65–67, where it is noted that the problem is widespread, that it tends to be ignored by teachers, and that staff should be alert to signs of it occurring such that they may be in a position to deal firmly with it, backed by appropriate sanctions and procedures. The systems to detect bullying should be a part of the wider systems for detecting, monitoring and resolving undesirable behaviour generally. Bullying has received particular attention in the recognition of good practice in that the headteacher should take 'all reasonable and proper steps to prevent any of the pupils in his care from suffering injury from the actions of fellow pupils', and where pupils suffer some particular vulnerability the duty owed to that pupil is commensurately greater. The procedures to be adopted as good practice are set out in DfEE Circular 8/94, 'Pupil Behaviour and Discipline', which states:

> Bullying or other forms of harassment can make pupils' lives unhappy, can hinder their academic progress, and can sometimes push otherwise studious students into truancy . . . . School staff must be alert to signs of bullying and act promptly and firmly against it. Failure to respond to incidents may be interpreted as condoning the behaviour.
>
> (Circular 8/94, paras 55 and 56)

In so far as DfEE Circulars constitute 'plainly sensible advice', they are, arguably, the professional standard by which the actions of reasonable teachers, headteachers and LEAs will be guided. Failure to act on such guidance or to consider it carefully before taking another course of action makes any other response to bullying, including ignoring it, unprofessional.

Legislation and workplace bullying

Although there are differences between countries, perhaps best exemplified by the common law jurisdictions of Australia, America and Canada in comparison with the civil law minefield of Europe, this section examines consistent themes which are illustrated by international legal consideration. The law does respond to workplace bullying differently around the world, but lay people and victims in particular are more concerned with justice being done than the complex legal structures that underpin it.

This complexity is immediately obvious from a brief examination of the range of UK and EU laws which can be related to workplace bullying and its effects. This range includes the 1996 Employment Rights Act which has been used in respect of unfair dismissal and breaches of mutual trust and confidence. The Sex Discrimination Act 1975 deals with the practice of negative discrimination on the grounds of gender leading to the dismissal of an employee, or other detriment. Racial discrimination leading to dismissal is covered by the Race Relations Act 1976, and the Disability Discrimination Act 1995 provides the same degree of legal protection for people with disabilities or perceived disabilities.

Serious overt aggression, including the intentional harassment of employees by threatening, abusive or insulting words or behaviour, can be prosecuted under the Criminal Justice and Public Order Act 1944, whilst the civil and criminal provisions now in force under the Protection from Harassment Act 1996 cover intentional harassment, including stalking.

Whistle blowing, ever an antecedent of much adult bullying, gets some protection from the law under the Trade Union Reform and Employment Act 1993, with particular reference to health and safety issues, and the Public Interest Disclosures Act 1998, for cases of dismissal, redundancy or other detriment arising from acts of disclosure in the public interest. Field (1997) provides some brief guidance on the relevance of this legislation to particular examples of workplace bullying.

European law is still evolving; in particular the 1991 European Recommendation on Dignity at Work deals primarily with harassment. It is useful in that it recognises that protection should be provided by employers to particularly vulnerable groups often subject to bullying. These include young employees, those newly appointed, gay staff, ethnic minorities and those with disabilities. In addition, there is a statutory framework concerning health and safety issues arising out of European directives and set out in Management of Health and Safety at Work Regulations and implemented by the Health and Safety Executive (1992).

In the US the legal framework hinges on the concept of the 'hostile work environment', where typically it may have been made clear to an employee that continuation in employment may illegally be contingent upon sexual favours, but the courts allow that the hostile environment can result from abusive comments, offensive jokes, or visible pornography. A recent decision by the United States Court of Appeals for the Sixth Circuit highlights the fact that a hostile work environment that violates the law does not have to be based on sexual harassment. In this case, the court held that a hostile environment age discrimination case could be brought under the Age Discrimination in Employment Act. Usually, to establish such a claim, the employee must show that the harassment was based on age and that it unreasonably interfered with work performance and created an objectively intimidating, hostile, or offensive work environment. Accordingly, US-based employers who seek to avoid a hostile environment must not just guard against sexual harassment, they must also be seen to try to prevent a hostile environment based on age, religion, race, national origin, disability, etc. Just as sexual jokes can create a hostile environment, so can ethnic jokes. In this regard, it should be noted that two black employees filed a suit against their employer, alleging that the firm created a hostile environment by permitting e-mail to be transmitted that contained vile and offensive racial remarks. According to these employees, when they complained about the e-mail, they were threatened with demotion and termination.

It is important to understand that no particular body of legislation deals with workplace bullying or its consequences. A particular incident may be covered by several different laws; another incident may be covered by none of them. It is necessary to assess each situation carefully before deciding what, if any, legal action can be taken. The decisions made depend on what the claimants want; some may want a simple apology and the promise that they will be protected in the future; others may want compensation for post-traumatic stress effects and/or physical injury and have no intention of returning to their workplace. Many will seek compensation for unfair dismissal and want their job back, dignity restored and their position vindicated.

Employers and personal harassment policies and practices

In general terms, it is apparent that the employment legislation of most developed countries provides a measure of protection to victims, although the pathways to this protection may be different. In the UK, responsibilities of employers are clearly delineated; they do have a duty of care to their employees and should be proactive in ensuring that this duty is met. A considerable amount of guidance has been provided to assist employers in formulating appropriate policies and strategies in order to establish workplace environments that are safe. This guidance can be broadly summarised to provide a context in which the antecedents, the harassing behaviour and the consequences to victims and workplace environment can be assessed.

In the first place, employees should be made aware that harassment of all types is unacceptable and may lead to disciplinary action. The range of behaviours considered to be harassing should be identified to include the types of problems experienced by victims of workplace bullying, ranging from physical assault to rumour-mongering and intimidation. The written material should state what steps will be taken if there are problems reported and there should be clear guidance as to the way in which victims can report bullying.

Employers should establish clear investigatory and disciplinary procedures. Ideally sanctions should be available for consistent use so that there is a uniform response to bullying which may lead to dismissal. This is a very important aspect of policy because some employees who are dismissed or otherwise sanctioned for bullying may claim that their treatment has been unfair if such sanctions have not been used consistently in previous cases that are similar.

Investigations should consider carefully any mitigating factors that may exist or be claimed. These may well include evidence about the victim's behaviour which was perceived to be provocative or irritating. Factors about the workplace environment or the organisation of the work may be relevant. Where issues of disruption, inappropriate behaviour and work practices and inadequate management are identified then steps must be seen to be taken to correct them. If disciplinary action is taken against any individual there is an expectation that this will be fully documented in records giving also the reasons derived from the investigation.

As is often the case, legislation and the guidance which accompanies it seek to encourage good practice by reinforcing it and using it as a model. In theory, at least, employers are encouraged to create workplace environments that are inimical to the development of bullying behaviours. In part, therefore, the legal position on workplace bullying is to hold the employer responsible for allowing a working environment where bullying flourished. The direct perpetrators themselves are seldom on trial unless their behaviour has constituted a breach of criminal law. Often, their excuse is that they were unaware of the serious consequences of their activities or they were only teasing the victim who they claim was too sensitive and should have been able to take a joke. Such rationalisations are irrelevant; if the employer can be shown to have permitted the behaviour by not taking preventative steps then the victim may have a case.

Although the earlier history of such cases was predominantly associated with racial and sexual harassment, the present-day situation is broad and becoming clearer. EU law, particularly, adopts a broad-brush approach and the European Recommendation of Dignity at Work (1991) extends protection well beyond the early boundaries. In addition, it provides a code of practice for employers to adopt and modify to suit their particular needs and organisation. This Recommendation reinforces the view that freedom from oppression and intimidation in the workplace is the right of all employees and it is the duty of management to secure this right. It is not the right of management to allow or reward a workplace culture based on harassment and fear on the grounds that this is a valid management style for getting things done. Whether or not managers and employers consider bullying to be a natural pattern of some relationships – the unpleasant humour of pranksters or the just deserts of provocative victims – makes no difference if these behaviours are unwanted by the victims and inimical to their welfare. The code of the Recommendation is there as a standard to be reached by employers, and failure to do so can be judged accordingly in courts and tribunals throughout the EU.

Mobbing and legal issues

The definition of mobbing provides a useful starting point for analysis of particular cases of workplace bullying. Leymann's (1996) definition may be used as a basis of investigation about the nature of individual cases. Mobbing has been conceptualised as showing itself in three formats: (a) by employees against a colleague; (b) by employees against a subordinate; (c) by employees against their line manager. These are sometimes referred to as horizontal, downward and upward mobbing (Ramage, 1996). Ramage makes the point, that whatever its direction, mobbing has characteristics which lead often to claims of constructive dismissal; for example, because of lack of support given to the employees by their employers. The employees believe that they can only escape the mobbing by leaving their employment. Sometimes the effect on the victim's health is so great that their performance suffers and they are either sacked or asked to resign.

A classic example of 'horizontal' mobbing was reported in the UK press on 20 February 2000. This case was of a 33-year-old machinist in a West Yorkshire plastics factory who allegedly became a 'punchbag' when his colleagues found that he was illiterate through dyslexia. On several occasions he was trussed up in shrink-wrap plastic and once felt that he nearly suffocated because of this.

He told the press: 'I hated working there but I had to stay because I have a young family and needed the money.' This victim suffered sleeplessness and depression; his relationship with his partner and their children deteriorated. Eventually he walked out of the job. The case went before a tribunal in Leeds where the victim was awarded a then record sum of £28,000 for what was described as 'a rather extreme case of barbarous treatment'. Apparently the victim had complained to the management on several occasions but was simply ignored. There was no investigation. As a consequence the tribunal ruled that he had been unfairly dismissed and also discriminated against on the basis of disability. The tribunal warned that although such behaviour was accepted at one time in the workplace, it has now been outlawed. Employees and employers were advised to heed this fact.

In most cases of horizontal mobbing the victim's probable course of action is likely to be a claim of constructive dismissal. There are problems which face such an action. These include:

- showing that there was a breach of contract in that there had been a failure of the duty of care;
- showing that there actually had been workplace bullying by more than one colleague. It is necessary to show what had been done and by whom on how many occasions;
- showing that the allegations of the victim are more likely to be true than the denials of the perpetrators;

- showing that the employer is vicariously liable for the behaviour of the perpetrators. This means showing that these behaviours occurred during the course of employment when the employees were doing what they were supposed to be doing.

The ways in which the employer deals with workplace bullying are of crucial importance. One way in which the employer can defend himself is by showing that he or she has a good system for monitoring and supervising the behaviour of staff. If such a system exists but the employer has not made adequate use of it, then the victim has a case for constructive dismissal. This situation would be a breach of the duty of care and represents an undermining of the mutual duty of trust.

The employee must have made recorded attempts to engage the support of the employer. It must be shown that the employer knew or should have known of the behaviour. If this is the case, the employer cannot state that he or she was unaware of the harassment. The employer is supposed to have systems for supervising and monitoring what employees are doing during the course of their working hours. Failure to have a satisfactory means of supervising makes the employer vulnerable to legal action in the case of mobbing. If, however, the employer has reasonable methods of supervision in place but the victim has still been subject to bullying, then questions will be asked as to whether the victim has attempted to inform the employer of the problems.

Examples of downward mobbing are often found when there is a concerted effort to get rid of an older employee or a person of an ethnic minority. Examples of upward mobbing are not common in the legal arena; few managers dare to admit that they are being bullied by their staff. One area where there are fewer reservations of this sort is that of sexual harassment which is fairly well protected by law (see above). Employees can bully a line manager in a wide variety of ways. One of the most common is to contrive to make him or her look incompetent by withholding information. Systematic failure to carry out jobs efficiently, such that the line manager is taken to task by superiors for failing to meet targets, is also frequent.

Particularly severe cases have been known where the line manager's computer data storage is sabotaged and important work is lost. Another common strategy is to start rumours about the morals of the line manager; sexual slurs, hints of drug or alcohol abuse and tales of disloyalty to the employer quickly do the rounds and damage the line manager's reputation and credibility.

As may be seen, the victims of this form of mobbing are in a weak position; if they complain to their own managers then they may become suspect as poor leaders and unsuitable for their positions. The more senior the manager, the more difficult it is for them to seek support from above. Paradoxically, failure to report what is happening means that the manager appears unwilling to take up procedures the employer has for stopping workplace bullying. As has been shown above, this places the victim's legal position in jeopardy.

The need for accurate assessment

The complexities of workplace bullying and the associated employment legislation make necessary an adequate means of assessing individual cases and a sufficiently robust model to guide assessment. The need for full assessment becomes even greater in the UK now that the Human Rights Act 2000 is established. Quite what impact this will have on the number of litigations arising from bullying is not yet clear, although predictions are generally that there will be an increase. Without adequate assessment there is little prospect of bullied employees and their employers benefiting from the legal opportunities affording protection. The next chapter provides models of workplace bullying and places the behaviour within the more general domain of human aggression. This allows for a partitioning of the principal ante-cedents, subsequent bullying behaviour and its consequences for accurate investigation.

Chapter 2

Workplace bullying as a variety of human aggression

The relativities of workplace bullying to the more general subject of human aggression are not ones that have been researched extensively and, indeed, much of the literature on both school-based and workplace bullying unwittingly or otherwise portrays bullying as a unique phenomenon that is largely context-specific. Yet even when particular paradigms of aggression are examined closely there will be found parallels that are easily overlooked because of adherence to context specificity. This limitation has parallels in other areas of the study of aggression; for example, the gross differences claimed between human and animal aggression which continue to prevent serious attempts at syntheses (Blanchard, Herbert and Blanchard, 1999). Despite the fact that varieties of aggression have obvious similarities between human and non-human species in that both show offensive attack, defensive attack, play-fighting and predation (of which, perhaps, bullying is a notable human example), there is reluctance to find unifying theories or explanatory models to further research. Similarly, there appears to be a reluctance to view adult bullying as another example of the aggression that humans can inflict on each other.

For example, war is often held to be the most dramatic and devastating form of human aggression in that one human can, with a press of a button, cause untold devastation and loss of life. On the face of it, there seems little similarity between such culturally and politically induced aggression on a mass scale and the vicious subjugation of underlings practised by a bullying line manager. Yet it must be remembered that even within the arena of war there are gross individual differences between participants. Thus, one victorious commanding officer may take prisoners and treat them well whilst another may practise rape, torture and further a programme of genocide. Although this is a crude comparison, there are to be found in the many forms of politically induced engagement called war examples of those who progress to the point of meeting their objectives and those who, like bullies in the workplace or schools, may go beyond mission objectives, in the pursuit of individual gratification, bringing rape, torture and genocide to their victims.

A major theme of this book is that the proper study of bullying, in the workplace and other contexts, is within the research arena of human aggression. This is not an original contention; some others who have researched workplace aggression (e.g, Baron and Neuman 1996; Baron, Neuman and Geddes, 1999) have also pursued such a linkage robustly, and it is noteworthy that Brodsky (1976) considered that harassment in the workplace is intrinsic to the human condition and would always occur. It can be argued that since most theories of aggression come from experimental psychology, where research design has often contrived situations whereby strangers aggress against each other (e.g. Geen, 1990), this minimises their usefulness to the study of bullying in contexts where individuals know each other and modify their interpersonal behaviour accordingly (Hoel, Rayner and Cooper, 1999).

One of the many difficulties encountered in the study of workplace bullying as a subset of human aggressive behaviours is that the term 'aggression' is one of the most value-laden when applied to human behaviour and is at the same time one of the least well defined for the purposes of operation definition in research. For example, Benjamin (1985) likened it to 'intelligence' and 'self-esteem' as particular examples to demonstrate the difficulties of conceptual analysis. In addition, Hoel *et al.* (1999) point out that the majority of studies of human aggression are limited, being focused mainly on affective rather than instrumental aggression. As has been pointed out previously (Randall, 1997a), bullying can fulfil the criteria for either or both independently of the nature and context of specific incidents.

There had been many attempts at formulating unifying theories of human aggression throughout the long period of research into this phenomenon. Early views took a biological stance in suggesting that aggression arose as part of a biological predisposition (e.g. Lorenz, 1966) or simply as a behavioural act (e.g. Buss, 1961) which could be studied independently of those involved in the behaviour and the setting in which it occurred. As limiting as the latter appears within the context of workplace aggression, Buss (1961) did provide a categorisation of human aggressive behaviour which has been made useful by later researchers (e.g. Baron and Neuman, 1996); further description of this will be given in a later section of this chapter. The role of frustration as an eliciting stimulus was given prominence by Dollard, Doob, Miller, Mowrer and Sears (1939) in the formulation of their frustration-aggression hypothesis, and this has also been used as part of a stress hypothesis for aggression (e.g. Berkowitz, 1989). Geen (1990) considered that the role of environmental factors in eliciting aggressive behaviour was, perhaps, more important than the learning of such behaviour through social learning theory. Emphasis is placed on the dynamic factors that link characteristic traits of people involved in particular aggressive encounters, the situation in which this occurs and the cognitive processes that mediate the interaction.

Cox and Leather (1994) took this viewpoint further by attempting to apply a cognitive behavioural theory of aggression to the concept of workplace violence. In their view, aggression is a coping response or a problem-solving approach to frustrations arising within the work context. Thus aggression is interpreted in the light of the subjective perceptions of the people involved in aggressive interactions which they interpret according to their own values and expectations. In evaluating the relationship between factors occurring in the workplace such as stress and workplace bullying, Einarsen, Raknes and Matthiesen (1994) point out that both bullies and victims should take part in a study where both levels of stress and bullying are measured. Logically if a stress-based hypothesis (e.g. Berkowitz, 1989) is valid, bullies should be identified as having particularly high levels of stress, whilst social inter-actionist models would predict higher levels of stress for victims. It is obvious, however, that neither of these findings is mutually exclusive. There is no reason why bullies should not respond to a level of stress by bullying and victims respond to the same stressful workplace environments and the impact of the bullying by becoming even more stressed than they were.

It is inevitable that human aggression can only be viewed as a social behavioural phenomenon since it cannot occur in any other setting. Baron (1997) stated that aggression 'stems from aspects of the social environment that instigated its occurrence and influenced both its form and direction' (p.122). Social interactionist theories of aggression are therefore helpful as a means of explaining aggressive behaviour. Thus, Felson and Tedeschi (1993) and Leather and Lawrence (1995) emphasise the importance of interpersonal influences throughout conflict situations and pay particular attention to the interaction between individuals. Felson (1992) states that external factors may elicit violations of social rules and may have more importance than the psychological characteristics of the individuals involved. As such, bullying becomes an intentional response to these external conditions and is used as a means of controlling them. This resonates well with clinical narrative studies of incidents of bullying that have clearly been used for the purposes of social control within particular contexts (e.g. Randall, 1997).

The issue of intention is not particular to the study of workplace bullying. Siann (1985) suggested that four conditions set the criteria for a behaviour that can be described as aggressive. These criteria are:

1   The aggressor *intends* to carry out the behaviour.
2   The behaviour takes place within inter-personal contexts that include conflict or competition.
3   The behaviour is *intended* to gain some advantage over the victim.
4   The aggressor should have either provoked the aggressive incident or intensified it.

Siann does not limit this set of criteria to physical violence only and under-lines this by including those forms of human aggression that may culminate in the use of force of a physical nature known as 'violence'. This gradation is helpful but only within a restricted range of contexts.

Issues of intention are important also to the inter-personal context of aggression when retaliation is involved. People are more likely to retaliate aggressively if they perceive the intentions of the other person or people to be malicious (Zillmann, 1996) and Siann (1985) suggests that complex social judgements are made about the intentions and motives of the participants which are matched up to whatever is regarded as normal and expected in the particular social situation. Given that many workplace bullies excuse their behaviour on the grounds that they are responding only to a perceived threat (e.g. Randall, 1997a), it is likely that aggression escalates when responses are viewed as being excessively aggressive by one or other parties taking part in a particular conflict-based interaction (e.g. Cox and Leather, 1994). A number of factors influence the ways in which people make such judgements and these include both internal and external variables. Thus, conflict is likely to escalate if the personality of an individual is viewed negatively, if the actions of a person are perceived as stress-evoking, if there are particular influences on inhibitory controls such as alcohol or drugs and the presence of observers who might witness 'loss of face' (e.g. Randall, 1997a). Such influences may well constitute triggers for aggressive escalation, and a considerable variety of these triggers have been noted within the mass of research publications into workplace bullying.

The issue of intention is important also when considering aggressive responses to perceived provocation. Ferguson and Rule (1983) provided a set of three criteria which may be used by individuals making judgements as to whether or not an aggressive response is appropriate to a perceived provocation. They state that an aggressive reaction is more likely if individuals believe that the provocative behaviour was intentional. Ferguson and Rule provide some indicators for judging whether or not intention was present and these include judgements about whether other behaviours could have been used instead of provocative behaviour; consideration about the benefits to the provocative person of using that behaviour; the difficulty associated with the production of that behaviour; and the past history of the individual behaving in that way.

The second set of criteria concerns judgements about whether or not specified provocative behaviours were malevolent. Such behaviour is judged to be malevolent if there is some obvious benefit for the provocator at the expense of the victim and/or the provocative action is seen as retaliatory for some previous aggressive behaviour.

The final set of criteria concerns judgement as to whether or not the behaviour could have been predicted as likely to cause harm to the victim; this would include neglectful acts or behaviour which would put the victim at risk of physical harm. Examples of this in workplace situations are commonly encountered when a negligent worker leaves dangerous material or machinery unguarded or acts in such a way as to impede another person dangerously.

Obviously if certain behaviours are judged to be unintentional and have an unforeseeable outcome then it is unlikely that an aggressive response will ensue. If, however, the behaviour is judged to be both intentional and malevolent then an angry aggressive response is more likely to be directed at the perpetrator. If the perpetrator continues to act in this way then the level of aggressive response is liable to escalate and a response set of bullying could be established. These 'judgements' made about perceived provocation fit well within a cognitive-behavioural model of human aggression and may be regarded as internalised forms of stimulus control.

It is noteworthy that the social interactionist perspective does not preclude considerations of personality or individual differences. For example, some individuals who lack the confidence or social skills needed to resolve conflict through assertive means may well resort to covert aggressive strategies to achieve the same end (e.g. Tedeschi, 1983). Dodge, Price, Bachorowski and Newman (1990) speak of a 'hostility attributional bias' which is the tendency to assume that apparently provocative behaviour from others is intentional and malevolent. People who are subjected to this bias are, therefore, more likely to respond aggressively rapidly in response to perceived provocation.

Another major theory of human aggression is that derived from social learning theory which describes the role of learning in social development generally. Its most famous proposer, Bandura (1978), has applied it robustly to the development of human aggression to explain how aggressive behaviours become assimilated, and how they are elicited and maintained. With specific reference to the development of aggressive behaviour, Bandura demonstrated (1977) that people learn to behave aggressively because they perceive that it is not only acceptable in some contexts but is also reinforced positively. Social learning theory states that individuals do not necessarily, in the first instance, need to experience this result for themselves but merely witness reinforcement occurring to others as a result of their aggressive behaviour. It has also been proposed that the mass-media portrayals of aggressive behaviour leading to positive reinforcement may also be sufficient models for the development of aggressive behaviour in young people (e.g. Aluja-Fabregat and Torrubia-Beltri, 1998). The perceived reinforcement of aggressive behaviour is the central plank of social learning theory. If individuals do not perceive aggressive behaviour reinforced, then Bandura proposes that they might identify other forms of behaviour with whatever eliciting stimuli are present. It is easy to conceptualise positive reinforcement in terms of a direct gain by aggressors, but more subtle reinforcers can exist in terms of the use of aggression to prevent some aversive event from occurring or for the purposes of causing some aversive events to cease (negative reinforcement).

Bandura (1983) also presents the other side of the coin by stating that the experience of aggression being sanctioned and rejected leads to a reduced potential for producing such behaviour when similar stimuli occur. He suggests that individuals will then experience disapproval by self of their own behaviour which is an aversive event of self-sanction.

Although not explicit to statement of social learning theory, it is clear that sets of circumstances which in some way erode the capacity of an individual for self-sanction may lead to a raised probability of aggressive behaviour. One variable which is commented upon frequently in the relevant literature is anonymity; for example, Zimbardo (1970) described the process of 'deindividuation' which is a diminution of the individual's monitoring of his/her social behaviour due to a perceived reduction in the way in which other people perceive them. Put crudely, this theory places in psychological terminology the commonly held belief that some people will engage in undesirable behaviour (including aggression) when they feel that they are unlikely to be identified. This resonates well with the concept of an 'effect–danger' ratio (Bjorkqvist, Osterman and Largerspetz, 1994) and the variety of cost-benefits analyses important to social exchange theory (e.g. Frude, 1992).

Zimbardo (1970) identifies other ways in which this process can occur, such as being a member of a group, which increases anonymity and proportions blame, responsibility and guilt over a greater number of people.

Group membership is thought also to lead to a weakening of individuals' inhibitions of behaviour where the rules of social behaviour in the particular context are not clear. The common example used is of the football supporter whose aggressive behaviour is increased in a crowd of fans but not in other contexts. Another common example quoted is of individuals who succumb to the influence of alcohol or drugs and whose individual capacity for behavioural self-monitoring becomes diminished.

It is apparent that this theory of aggressive behaviour forms one bridge between the social interactionists' perspective which emphasises 'guidance' afforded by particular environmental contexts, and social learning theory which emphasises the role of positive reinforcement or perceived positive reinforcement. Clearly, where social behaviour is less constrained than is normal (e.g. as in a crowd of football supporters as opposed to other community settings), then that context provides a setting in which individuals may relax their self-monitoring. In this way, aggressive behaviour can be shown to have both external and internal mediators.

The example of an individual functioning within a football crowd is apposite also to considerations of the effect of arousal on aggressive behaviour. The frustration/aggression hypothesis propounded by Dollard and colleagues in 1939 has long since been held to be too simplistic and it is evident that other stimuli are just as potent in eliciting aggressive behaviour. The group arousal of football fans, particularly when confronted with the fans of the opposition, is observed to lead to increased rates of aggressive behaviour.

Justification for the subsequent conflicts, is then sought frequently by reference to the process of 'scapegoating' described by Schachter and Singer (1962). Scapegoating becomes a cognitive mechanism for ascribing blame to others in order to diminish responsibilities for one's own aggressive behaviour. To this complex brew of external and internal mediators of aggression may be added the effects of excessive alcohol.

Finally, this consideration of human aggression would not be complete without reference to relevant factors of the physical environment in which aggression may occur. It is apparent that there may be many context-specific factors relating to particular workplace situations that give rise to stress or frustration and which may then elicit aggressive responses. Amongst the most common and best-researched are the effects of heat, crowding and noise (e.g. Anderson, Anderson and Deuser, 1996). Bell (1981) showed that the incidence of aggressive behaviour rises as temperature rises until a point is reached where further increases of temperature are associated with reduced aggressive behaviour. Worchel and Teddlie (1976) found that perceived invasion of personal space can result in aggressive responses and noisy environments are found to produce higher levels of aggressive behaviour than quiet ones (Neuman and Baron, 1998).

Linking workplace bullying to human aggression

Randall (1997) demonstrated how behaviours subsumed under the label of 'bullying' can be aligned with the operational definitions of instrumental and affective aggression. Affective aggression is that which is accompanied by strong negative emotions, and anger is the particular emotional state which is considered to stimulate aggressive behaviour by acting as an intervening setting condition which at first initiates and then guides and maintains aggressive behaviour. Aggression theory has it that anger is evoked by some provocative stimulus or stimuli and the subsequent aggression is aimed at causing injury or other harm to the provocator (Feshbach, 1964). This form of aggression is instantly recognisable to the aggressor because of the associated changes in central and autonomic nervous systems activity, causing increased blood flow to the musculature, a rise in blood pressure and pulse rate, a diminished flow of blood to the viscera and dilation of the pupils (Randall, 1997a).

Berkowitz (1983) argues that aggression need not necessarily be motivated by anger or another strong negative emotion. His theory of human aggression conceptualises a potentially large associative network in which emotions, dispositions and cognitions associated with aggressive behaviour may be stimulated by other factors with which they are closely linked. The concept of instrumental aggression arises from this and is exemplified by warfare between nations and the maintenance of power over targeted people (Tedeschi, 1983). The kind of bullying experienced by victims of their line manager is often related to the maintenance of power, and most bullying contexts involve an imbalance of power in favour of the aggressor. Olwcus (1993) makes the point that whatever else may be true of bullying there is always an imbalance of power.

The range of aggressive behaviours that fall within the concepts of affective and instrumental aggression is very considerable and, in respect of workplace contexts, Keashly (1998) identifies the difficulty of describing or observing subtle forms of aggression such as a 'harsh tone' or sarcasm. She points to the work of Baron and Neuman (1996) where they utilised the framework provided by Buss (1961) for categorising human aggression. As described in Chapter 1, Baron and Neuman identify the behaviour that Scandinavian and UK researchers call 'workplace bullying' as 'workplace aggression', and in making use of the Buss categorisation of human aggression they not only make possible more refined description and observation of subtle forms of aggression but also link directly workplace aggression/ workplace bullying to the more general research domain and literature of human aggression. In describing a major theme of their research they state:

> Workplace aggression is, in the final analysis, human aggression occurring in a specific context – the varied locations where people work. Since conditions in workplaces are, in some respect, unique (e.g. Employees interact with one another more frequently and over longer periods of time than is true of many other social settings), some of the variables that influence workplace aggression too, may be unique. However, it is our view that many of the factors that have been found to influence human aggression generally may also play a role in the occurrence in workplace aggression.
>
> (Neuman and Baron, 1998, p. 413)

Given this theme, they argue that a primary task for researchers of workplace aggression/workplace bullying should be that of the building of conceptual and empirical links between ongoing research and the existing literature concerning human aggression. Correctly, they state that this is not only a requirement of good scientific method but is also the best way of coming to understand properly and manage this aversive behaviour.

Clinical narrative studies (e.g. Randall, 1997, 1996) indicate that, at both the child and adult level, bullies tend to pick forms of bullying or locations for bullying that protect them from discovery by more powerful others. These findings support the earlier work of Bjorkqvist and her colleagues who introduced the concept of an effect–danger ratio which suggests that aggressors generally choose aggressive behaviours that are effective in harming the victim, while at the same time bringing about as little risk to themselves as possible. There are sex differences to be found within this practice amongst adults (Bjorkqvist, Osterman and Largerspetz, 1994, abstract A), as found in a study of 338 university employees (162 males, 176 females) who completed the Work Harassment Scale devised by Bjorkqvist and her colleagues (1994, abstract B). It was found that men were more likely to use rational-appearing aggression whilst women were more likely to use social manipulation. Both are variants of overt aggression used by perpetrators who are trying to disguise their aggressive intentions in order to avoid condemnation or retaliation.The effect–danger ratio is a reference to the subjective estimation of aggressors before displaying aggressive behaviour. Clinical study (e.g. Randall, 1997) suggests that aggressors perpetrating workplace bullying endeavour to maximise the effect of their behaviour whilst minimising the risk to themselves.

In more recent research Bjorkqvist and colleagues have demonstrated that the variables of empathy and social intelligence limit the degree to which direct aggressive behaviour is delivered. Thus Kaukiainen, Bjorkqvist, Largerspetz Osterman, Salmivalli, Rothberg and Ahlbom (1999) examined 526 Finnish schoolchildren from 10 to 14 years old and found that indirect aggression correlated positively and significantly with social intelligence in every age group studied. Thus those children who were the most socially intelligent were the most likely to use indirect forms of aggression. Physical and verbal forms of aggression had an almost zero correlation with social intelligence. Empathy correlated negatively and significantly with all types of aggression except indirect aggression in 12-year-old children. These findings suggest that children with good social intelligence use this as a means of maximising the effect/danger ratio in their favour, whilst those with high levels of empathy are less likely to use any form of aggression except, perhaps, indirect aggression in relation to the 12-year-old children studied.

Bjorkqvist, Osterman and Kaukiainen (2000) state that empathy reduces aggressive behaviour but social intelligence merely seems to limit its variety to indirect rather than direct forms. The researchers state that social intelligence is required for all types of conflict behaviour, pro-social as well as antisocial, but that empathy functions as a mitigator of aggression. The researchers believe that when the effects of empathy are partialled out, correlations between social intelligence and all types of aggression increase whereas correlations between social intelligence and non-aggressive conflict resolution decrease. It is clear, therefore, that social intelligence is related to various forms of aggressive behaviour; the strength of the relationship is greater in respect of indirect aggression and is weaker in respect of physical aggression. These findings accord well with the developmental theory of aggressive style (Bjorkqvist, Osterman and Kaukiainen, 2000). In addition there is a relationship to locus of control in that for boys (aged 11 to 15 years) physical, verbal and indirect forms of aggression are correlated significantly with external locus of control, whereas in girls no significant relationship between aggression and locus of control was found (Osterman, Bjorkqvist, Largerspetz, Charpentier, Caprara and Pastorelli, 1999).

Baron and Neuman (1996) point out that although the maximisation of the effect–danger ratio is invariably sought by aggressors in all contexts, there are factors about workplace environments which make this trend even stronger. First, people at work are often in repeated contact with each other during the course of the working day. As a consequence, would-be aggressors know that they are likely to be in repeated contact with their victims and observers of the aggression for the foreseeable future. The probability of retaliation is therefore increased, as is the likelihood of some other 'danger' emanating from observers who may take action against the aggressor. A number of studies (e.g. Rogers, 1980) demonstrate that the likelihood or anticipation of retaliation is an inhibitor of subsequent aggression, especially in its more overt form. Similarly, studies (e.g. Borden, 1975) demonstrate that overt aggression is reduced in the presence of observers, although this is not always the case in workplace bullying where observers may actually be supportive of bullies (Randall, 1997). Baron and Neuman (1996) hypothesise that these inhibitory factors cause would-be aggressors to function in ways which would be covert as opposed to overt in order to disguise their identity and/or true intentions.

In seeking to test the hypothesis that workplace aggression/bullying would be more likely to take the form of covert rather than overt aggression, Baron and Neuman turned to the framework of human aggression proposed by Buss (1961). This system categorises human aggression in terms of three dichotomies: verbal–physical, direct–indirect, and active–passive. These dichotomies are then subdivided according to whether the aggression is direct or indirect. Verbal forms consist of efforts to cause harm using words, whereas physical forms of aggression make use of overt actions to cause harm. Direct forms of aggression are those where harm is delivered directly to targets, whereas indirect forms inflict harm through the actions of other agents or on people, objects and/or resources that are valued by the target. Active aggressive forms cause harm through the performance of some behaviour, whereas passive forms cause the damage by withholding something valued by the victim.

Baron and Neuman present examples of these eight forms of aggression from the workplace context and predict that the most common form of aggression in the workplace would be verbal, passive and indirect rather than physical, active and direct. The eight examples they give range from failing to deny false rumours about the target (victim) as a form of verbal-passive-indirect aggression, through to physical attacks (e.g. pushing, shoving, hitting) or negative or obscene gestures towards the target, as examples of the physical-active-direct form.

Baron and Neuman also sought to examine whether increasing workplace stressors would bring about an elevation in workplace aggression frequency.

At the time of their study several research studies had examined what happened when particular stressors were increased. For example, Anderson, Deuser and DeNeve (1995) had reported on the effects on affective aggression of temperature, hostile affect, hostile cognition and arousal, and Berkowitz (1989) had revisited the frustration-aggression hypothesis. Diversity amongst employees was also found to be associated with increased negative attitudes towards organisations (Tsui, Egan and O'Reilly, 1994); and Konovsky and Brockner (1993) had written about the increase of negative cognitions, anxiety and frustration associated with the layoff of staff.

Baron and Neuman's study, therefore, attempted to determine the linkage between conventionally defined forms of human aggression and stimulus and setting factors specifically associated with the workplace. Contrary to expectation, however, the research findings suggested that direct actions were more frequent than indirect actions, although the first hypothesis was partly substantiated because participants reported that verbal and passive forms of aggression occurred more frequently in their workplace settings than physical and active forms. In discussing these results Baron and Neuman (1996) suggest that, while passive forms of aggression may prevent aggressor identification and victim retaliation, indirect forms are less effective in producing harm. As a consequence, passive forms would be more common in the workplace settings than active forms but indirect forms are less likely to be as frequent as direct forms.

A theoretical model of workplace aggression

In discussing the potential causes of aggression, Neuman and Baron (1998) provide a theoretical model of workplace aggression to facilitate the understanding of causation. They suggest that such a model may also be useful in formulating prevention strategies. The model they propose is shown in Figure 1 and the following sections summarise the constituent variables.

Their classification of these factors is based upon an assiduous review of the relevant literature and many of their conclusions are congruent with findings from Scandinavian research on workplace bullying.

Unfair treatment

Leaving aside severe instances of workplace violence, such as murder or attempted murder, there is a growing body of evidence that the perception of unfair treatment is associated with a variety of aggressive acts in the workplace. For example, Cropanzano and Baron (cited by Neuman and Baron, 1998) found that perception of unfair treatment is an antecedent to conflict. In addition, Neuman and Baron's own study (1997) stated that individuals who perceive themselves to have been treated unfairly by their line managers showed elevated occurrences of engaging in aggressive acts.

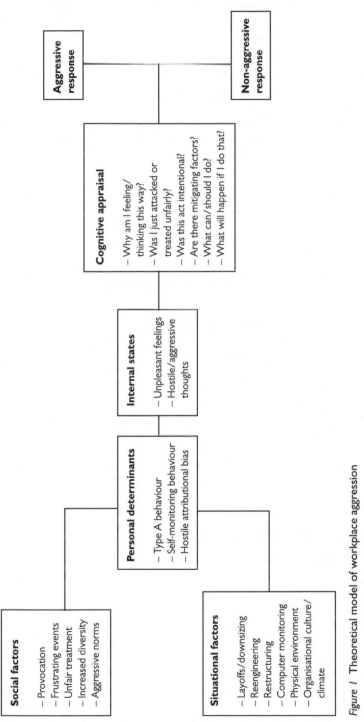

Figure 1 Theoretical model of workplace aggression
Source: Neuman and Baron, 1998, p. 401

Frustration-inducing events

The role of frustration as an elicitor of aggression has been described above. Neuman and Baron consider this to be a comparatively weak elicitor except in instances where individuals perceive that they are being thwarted deliberately and intentionally in an unfair manner (e.g. Geen, 1990). There is also a body of literature which indicates that frustrations perceived to be unfair are positively correlated with aggression directed at others and interference with production, stealing and other hostile acts (e.g. Storms and Spector, 1987).

Increased workforce diversity

Baron and Neuman refer to the literature which suggests that people are attracted to those who they believe are similar to themselves and repelled by others whom they believe to be different (e.g. Dryer and Horowitz, 1997). Neuman and Baron (1998) comment that these differences generate negative affect leading to an increased probability of aggression.

Normative behaviour and norm violations

Neuman and Baron (1998) present evidence that many workers believe that some forms of aggression are to be expected. Verbal abuse is under-reported because many workers expect it to occur as a normal aspect of job-related behaviour. There is growing evidence also that some organisations encourage hostility by allowing a conflictual workplace climate in which toughness is equated with an aggressive demeanour (e.g. Randall, 1997).

Neuman and Baron also present evidence that use of part-time and temporary contracts and job sharing are associated with workplace aggression, as is the failure of staff to keep within their own boundaries, particularly with regard to production work.

Situational determinants of aggression

Neuman and Baron (1998) make clear that this category includes situational and environmental contexts in which workplace aggression can occur. They employed two major subgroups, namely the **changing face of modern workplaces** and **environmental factors**.

With regard to the first of these, Neuman and Baron make use of research demonstrating the frustrating effects of redundancies, not only to those who are made redundant but also to those who witness what happens and experience stress and insecurity as well as resentment, depression and hostility. In respect of this, Neuman and Baron refer to the work of Catalano, Novaco and McConnell (1997) who extend frustration-aggression theory to hypothesise that an increasing frequency of redundancies has a countervailing influence on workplace aggression which is proportional to how many people lose their jobs in contrast to how many fear that their jobs will be lost. A theoretical model was put forward in this paper which estimates the net effect of these processes on the incidence of violence in the community and specifies a non-linear function in which small increases in redundancies are associated with increased frequency of aggression whereas large increases in redundancies are associated with reduced frequency. The authors claim that their model fits the data for both men and women.

Baron and Neuman are of the opinion also that forms of employee monitoring, particularly computer monitoring of productivity, are another situational variable associated with workplace aggression. For example, Smith and Carayon *et al.* (1992) used a questionnaire survey of employees in telecommunications companies to examine job stress in relation to the influence of electronic monitoring of job performance, satisfaction and employee health. Their questionnaire was returned by 745 employees from eight different companies, which was a response rate of approximately 25 per cent. Their results indicated that employees who have their performance monitored electronically experience their working conditions as more stressful and report higher levels of job boredom, psychological tension, depression, anxiety, health complaints, fatigue and anger than those who were not electronically monitored.

With regard to environmental conditions, Neuman and Baron include amongst these: high temperatures, high humidity, extreme cold, air quality and lighting. Crowding and high noise levels have also been linked to increased levels of aggression. Thus Anderson, Anderson and Deuser (1996) examined the effects of extreme temperatures on arousal, cognition and affect. As predicted, hot and cold temperatures increased state hostility and aggressive attitudes/thoughts. Cohn and Rotton (1997) found that time had a moderating effect on extremes of temperature as a mediator of aggression. They hypothesised that relations between temperature and assaults should be stronger during evening hours than during other hours of the day and tested this with an appropriate design using three-hour measures of assaults, temperature, and other weather variables for a two-year period. The hypothesis was confirmed and, in addition, assaults were found to decline after reaching a peak at moderately high temperatures. The probability of assaults was indeed found to increase during evening hours and also at weekends.

Personal determinants

In common with other researchers Neuman and Baron recognised that individuals have different propensities to aggression which are influenced by the social and situational factors outlined above. They identify three in particular as **Type A behaviour patterns, self-monitoring behaviour** and **hostile attributional bias**.

These are now considered in turn. Neuman and Baron (1998) make use of the time-honoured concept of the Type A individual. This type was first defined by Friedman and Rosenman in 1969 as individuals:

> who are engaged in a relatively chronic struggle to obtain an unlimited number of poorly defined things from their environment in the shortest period of time, and if necessary, against the opposing efforts of other things or persons in the same environment
>
> (cited by Jenkins, Zyzanski and Rosenman, 1979, p. 3)

Those individuals who exhibit the opposite type of behaviour, who are relaxed, mellow, unhurried and content, are designated Type B.

Type A individuals were described by Jenkins (1975) as having a behavioural syndrome or lifestyle that is characterised by extremes of competitiveness, striving for achievement, aggressiveness, haste, impatience, restlessness, explosiveness of speech, and feelings of being under pressure of time and workload (cited in Jenkins, Zyzanski and Rosenman, 1979). Elsewhere (e.g. Miller, Lack and Asroff, 1985) it has been indicated that Type A individuals want to control group situations and demonstrate higher levels of aggression than Type B individuals. Neuman and Baron (1997) identify the significant relationship between the Type A behaviour pattern and their closely specified forms of workplace aggression, expressions of hostility, obstructionism, and overt aggression. Thus they are more likely to direct their aggression against people whom they perceive to be satisfactory targets (e.g. Randall, 1997).

Consideration of the Type A behaviour pattern leads on to the issue of self-monitoring and its effects on the probability of aggressive behaviour. People with Type A patterns tend not to be very good at self-monitoring and find it hard to readily adjust their actions to changing circumstances. Snyder and Gangestad (1986) used a re-analysis of the results of the Self-Monitoring Scale to show that self-monitoring is a meaningful and interpretable causal variable having significant influences on social behaviour. Thus, people who are classified as high in self-monitoring behaviour are especially sensitive and modify their words and behaviours in order to create a favourable impression with others. Those who do not do this tend to be more conflictual and provocative in their behaviour, such that Neuman and Baron (1997) found a significant relationship between low self-monitoring and obstructionism.

With regard to hostility attributions, Neuman and Baron introduce this as a factor on the basis of findings that when individuals interpret other people's behaviour as hostile, they are more likely to feel aggrieved and retaliate. This is a well-researched finding; for example, Dodge and Coie (1987) studied hostility attributional effects amongst 259 elementary schoolchildren and found a strong influence of attributional bias on the manifestation of reactive aggressive behaviour during the course of free play.

Internal states and cognitive appraisal

Neuman and Baron make the commonsense point that feelings and thoughts are significant moderators of behaviour. They relate this to the appearance of human aggression in respect of **unpleasant feelings and hostile/aggressive thoughts** and **cognitive appraisal**. Clinical narratives abound with statements that unpleasant thoughts and negative moods are associated with increasing irritability and anger. In addition, aggression-related thoughts and memories are known to elicit unpleasant feelings and arousal. In brief, people who feel uncomfortable are more likely to show aggressive behaviour than those who do not. In organisational settings, the frustration induced by perceptions that treatment is intentional and unfair is positively correlated with aggression directed at others, interference with production, stealing and other hostile acts (e.g. Storms and Spector, 1987).

Finally, cognitive appraisal occurs before most acts of premeditated aggression. Mention has already been made of this appraisal in relation to the analysis carried out by potential aggressors in order to maximise harm whilst reducing damage to self.

The theoretical model of workplace bullying and learning theory

In formulating a model of workplace bullying within the domain of learning theories, a basic assumption is made that such aggressive behaviour is a sub-set of human aggression generally and is fashioned from the same set of developmental processes and range of antecedents and consequences. Whereas the workplace may provide unique stimulus control characteristics, these are assumed to act in much the same way in respect of aggressive behaviour as their counterparts in other domestic, community or institutional settings. The concept of stimulus control is employed within this model because it facilitates the linkage of developmental and personality factors with the more obvious organisational and infrastructural factors of the workplace. As variables included within general theories of learning as discriminative stimuli associated with the manifestations of specific behaviours, they enable eliciting factors to be linked to the concepts of positive and negative reinforcement which are important consequences able to maintain and/or strengthen behaviour.

This model enables a careful segmentation of the circumstances leading up to and maintaining the elevated risk of workplace bullying, and so affords a structure for investigation, assessment, amelioration and prevention. The subsequent chapters of this book then examine these sections and an attempt is made to incorporate material from the literature of other researchers (e.g. Baron and Neuman) and clinical practitioners.

Stimulus control

The concept of stimulus control is central to this model. This deals with learning to pay attention to, and eventually responding differentially to, events perceived in the environment (stimuli) that provide information about the effectiveness of behaviour, what behaviour is likely to be effective, the conditions under which it will be effective, and the likely consequences of that behaviour. According to operant learning theory, the consequences should take the form of positive and/or negative reinforcement which serves to maintain and/or strengthen the behaviour.

The effectiveness of particular discriminative stimuli (S^D) in the relationship between them, elicited behaviour and reinforcement (S^R), is determined by several independent parameters:

- the potency of the S^D, that is the strength with which they impinge on the recipient;
- the reliability of the S^D in predicting S^R, that is a function of the frequency with which these stimuli have been associated with reinforcement following the elicited behaviour;
- the immediacy of the S^R that the S^D predicts, that is, the more immediate the reinforcement, the more likely the behaviour is to be strengthened;
- the cost of attaining the S^R that the S^D predicts (e.g. the effect–danger ratio (explained by Bjorkqvist and her colleagues)).

Once a behaviour is strongly established by reinforcement it may thus achieve a degree of behavioural momentum which acts as a strong S^D even after environmental contingencies have changed. Thus, bullying which was once a response to a set of stimuli that provoked aggression may persist under its own momentum even after the original stimuli have been modified or terminated. Clinical studies (e.g. Randall, 1996) reveal this to be a common phenomenon in school-based bullying, where, for example, the original stimuli (e.g. a shift in friendship patterns within peer relations) are long forgotten.

This model of behavioural momentum explains how operant contingencies functioning within a strongly reinforcing environment will evoke behaviours that are resistant to extinction. This not only has implications for the difficulties confronting organisational change processes but also when dealing with individuals who need to recognise changes in environmental contingencies at the theoretical level. As Plaud and Plaud (1998) point out, this is one of the most fundamental goals of behaviour therapy. More specifically, it is such a goal also within cognitive-behavioural therapy during which both bullies and victims must alter their constructs about environmental contingencies in order to succeed.

A further behavioural concept which is related to this and which is of use in analysing bullying situations concerns role-governed behaviour, which is the 'natural product of human verbal behaviour' (Plaud and Plaud, 1998).

Role-governed behaviour is shaped by the cultural processes that define the ways in which society functions and enables behaviour to be demonstrated correctly without prior training. Such behaviour can also be shaped by sub-cultural processes and it is these that are potentially damaging. For example, attacks against ethnic minorities may be governed by local 'rules' which state what young people should do when in the presence of members of the minorities. Similarly, some victims may be the subject of 'rules' or constructs within an organisation or department which govern the way in which their colleagues respond to them. For example, one male victim was thought wrongly to have reported another worker for theft. In fact, it was the loss prevention officer for the firm who had made the accusation. Even when the situation became known the bullying did not stop, because a 'rule' had come into being which stated, 'This man must be punished.'

Some victims may assimilate the rules themselves and it is from this that self-contructs develop to the effect that 'I'm no good'. If these constructs develop sufficient strength then the victims may cut themselves off from positive reinforcement and suffer low self-esteem and even depression. Plaud and Newberry (1996) state that much of what is labelled as cognitive therapy involves changing the rule-governance of behaviour.

The interaction of operant and classical conditioning

Despite the commonplace separation of these two forms of learning during the conventional teaching of learning theory, operant and classical (Pavlovian) conditioning are normally components of integrated, seamless responses organisms make to their environment. In general, both are usually occurring during the output of daily behaviour and stimulus control variables constitute their interaction. The cyclic flow of behaviour and changes in the environment are generally so interwoven that classical and operant conditioning can only be acting together in a seamless evolution. Most particularly these two forms of conditioning unite in the way that stimuli come to control behaviour.

The interest in the interaction of classical and operant learning has captured the attention of learning theorists for decades (e.g. Hull, 1934). As mentioned above, arousal and other forms of proprioceptive stimuli are at the heart of the hypotheses about this interaction. This states that classically conditioned responses occur in operant learning, or alongside of it, because discriminative stimuli (S^D) are contingently paired to reinforcers in the presence of proprioceptive feedback. This is believed to increase the level of motivation, which further raises the probability that a behaviour will occur. The final shaping of that behaviour is, of course, directly linked to the experience of reinforcement following the behaviour, but the element of classical conditioning will serve to 'energise' it and so influence its intensity.

For example, a worker who is aware that a bullying person is approaching may find that his or her anticipatory response is augmented at the physiological level by unpleasant arousal. The strength of a particular avoidance response (e.g. going to the toilet or otherwise leaving the area) may indeed be elicited by the prospect of the negative reinforcement gained by 'turning off' the presence of the bully. The bodily sensation of arousal will tend to heighten the motivation for this behaviour and make it more likely to occur and more urgent when it does. Clearly, a therapeutic process for such a victim would need to take into account this additional 'energising' factor when attempting to gauge the strength of the response prior to replacing it with a more assertive behaviour. Another area where classical conditioning is of importance concerns the phenomenon of sign tracking whereby the individual monitors frequently the environment for 'signs' that an event is about to occur. In the workplace bullying situation, this is evident when a long-term victim constantly monitors the immediate environment for signs that his or her tormentor is about to appear. The following study provides a good example.

Richard, a 27-year-old leisure services administrator, alleged bullying by his line manager. 'I knew when she came into the reception area and I was there that she would start on me. She would look around at the registers, receipts and invoices that I had been working on and pick fault – endlessly. Our customers would be waiting to be served but it did not matter – she would still have a go. Then she would look at them with a big welcoming smile and say something like "He's a grand lad but I've got to keep helping him" as though I was a complete novice.

'If I could, I would get out of her way before she got to the reception area. I would listen for the whoosh of the double doors down the corridor from her office which, if it was her, would be followed by the squeak of the trainers she always wore. I listened for four squeaks if there was no one to be served. The whoosh followed by four squeaks meant that she would see my back through the glass of the last door. She couldn't say then that I had left reception unattended for ages.'

It is clear that this kind of tracking activity, which is a conditioned response (C^R) in terms of classical conditioning, will interrupt operant responses which are adaptive. Thus the worker who is constantly monitoring the environment for his or her tormentor cannot be fully engaged on task. Some learning theorists (e.g. Staddon, 1983) suggest that there is an interface between classical and operant learning prior to receipt of the terminal reinforcement. Thus, in the final linkage bullying behaviour is positively and/or negatively reinforced and so more likely to occur in the future as a consequence of operant processes. The intermediary behaviours which are reinforced only by the prospect of gaining the reinforcer can be regarded as conditioned responses to stimuli that signal the potential for reinforcement. In other words, each of these stimuli becomes a conditioned stimulus (C^S) with the potential to maintain a stream of behaviour.

Stimulus control variables associated with workplace bullying

The stimulus control variables associated with workplace bullying are drawn from both the European and American research on workplace bullying. There is a substantive degree of overlap and the categorisation of these variables according to their characteristics as Setting Stimuli, Setting Conditions, Internal States and Specific Events enables a linkage of these two important schools of thought. Figure 2 shows how these discriminative stimuli are associated with the elicitation of aggressive behaviour in the workplace and the consequent reinforcement of it.

These conceptualisations can be applied to victim behaviour as well as that of the aggressors. There is often a linkage of discriminative stimuli in the form of stimuli associated with the potential reinforcer. In the case of the young man above, the reinforcer is the reduction of stress associated with the incipient arrival of the bullying line manager which is 'signed' by the noises of opening doors and her shoes.

The example that follows (Figure 3) portrays a linkage in relation to the behaviour of an aggressive bully, and both operant and classical learning paradigms are at work.

This example can be dissected according to operant and classical theory. Functioning according to aggressive norms in the absence of direct reinforcement could be viewed as a C^S or as rule-governed behaviour with a prominence that is one of heavily reinforced operant behaviour. Such functioning reinforces the ready perception of provocation (S^R) and becomes the discriminative stimuli (S^D) for the expression of annoyance and/or anger.

The presence of peers who also subscribe to the aggressive norms of the organisation acts as reinforcing stimuli (S^R) for this expression and also as confirming discriminative stimuli (S^D) for the next step in the behavioural chain which, in this example, is the cognitive-behavioural response of hostility attribution which elevates arousal.

At this point in the example the aggressor considers factors associated with the effect–danger ratio. Victim traits are an important aspect of this calculation. A perception of the potential victim as annoying, complaining and less strong than the aggressor acts as reinforcing stimuli (S^R) for attribution and arousal and discriminative stimuli (S^D) for aggressive behaviour. The victim's

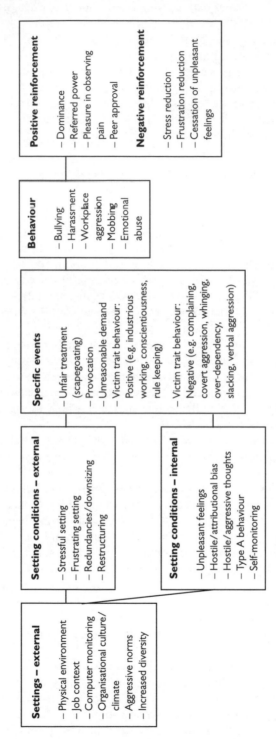

Settings – external

– Physical environment
– Job context
– Computer monitoring
– Organisational culture/
  climate
– Aggressive norms
– Increased diversity

Setting conditions – external

– Stressful setting
– Frustrating setting
– Redundancies/downsizing
– Restructuring

Setting conditions – internal

– Unpleasant feelings
– Hostile/attributional bias
– Hostile/aggressive thoughts
– Type A behaviour
– Self-monitoring

Specific events

– Unfair treatment
  (scapegoating)
– Provocation
– Unreasonable demand
– Victim trait behaviour:
  Positive (e.g. industrious
  working, conscientiousness,
  rule keeping)

– Victim trait behaviour:
  Negative (e.g. complaining,
  covert aggression, whinging,
  over-dependency,
  slacking, verbal aggression)

Behaviour

– Bullying
– Harassment
– Workplace
  aggression
– Mobbing
– Emotional
  abuse

Positive reinforcement

– Dominance
– Referred power
– Pleasure in observing
  pain
– Peer approval

Negative reinforcement

– Stress reduction
– Frustration reduction
– Cessation of unpleasant
  feelings

Figure 2 An antecedents–behaviour–consequences model of workplace bullying

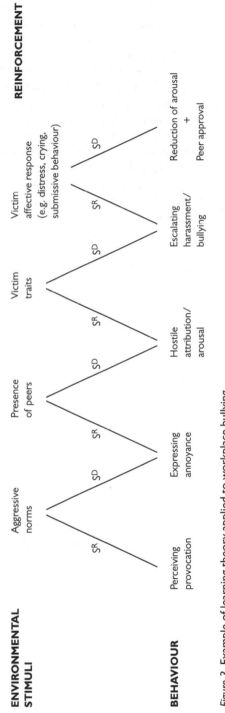

ENVIRONMENTAL STIMULI

Aggressive norms

Presence of peers

Victim traits

Victim affective response (e.g. distress, crying, submissive behaviour)

REINFORCEMENT

BEHAVIOUR

Perceiving provocation

Expressing annoyance

Hostile attribution/ arousal

Escalating harassment/ bullying

Reduction of arousal
+
Peer approval

S^R   S^D   S^R   S^D   S^R   S^D   S^R   S^D

Figure 3 Example of learning theory applied to workplace bullying

distressed behaviour provides reinforcement (S^R) in two ways. The reduction of the aggressor's arousal is a form of negative reinforcement and peer approval acts as a positive reinforcement.

Analysis of this sort enables the model of process to facilitate the investigation and amelioration of most incidents of workplace bullying. The analysis can be superimposed on the theoretical model depicted in Figure 2. Given that many of the constituent variables (e.g. physical environment) have been discussed already, the subsequent chapters provide a review of the traits of victims and bullies that are antecedents if not causes of workplace bullying. The next chapter, however, deals with the investigative aspects of assessment which are guided by the model in a stepwise examination of the antecedent conditions, the nature of the bullying behaviour and its consequences.

Chapter 3

A framework for assessment

Forensic psychological assessments are an increasingly important aspect of litigation. Traditionally, this has mainly involved the criminal domain of law where there have been concerns about competency to confess or to be put on trial, the nature of sentencing and the possibility of legal insanity used as a mitigation. Increasingly, the role of substance abuse has exercised many forensic psychologists, but a major area of growth concerns workers' claims for compensation for physical and psychological injury. Associated with the growth in this area has been a developing need for expert psychological assessments in relation to various forms of discrimination and the failure of employers in their duty of care.

As in most areas of psychological evaluation, this form of forensic examination has developed on the basis of a long-standing professional requirement for careful and thorough investigation of the difficulties experienced by clients or those difficulties they have created themselves. It is often the case that the assessments are not used solely for purposes of litigation but are also useful in identifying therapeutic needs and setting a benchmark from which therapeutic change can be evaluated. The clinical significance of forensic assessments cannot be underestimated and the need for painstaking evaluation as essential to the identification of remedial strategies has been described thoroughly (e.g. Matarazzo, 1983).

Within a clinical framework there are normally two major stages in the assessment of clients with presenting problems. The first stage is often referred to as the Information-Gathering Model (Finn and Tonsager, 1997) and is a comprehensive evaluation from which the clinician endeavours to evolve a hypothesis about the causes and maintenance of the presenting problems. This hypothesis is based not only on the clinician's experience of the client and whatever methods have been used to gain information but also on relevant psychological theory and research outcomes which link the individual assessment to the body of psychology that is most appropriate to the presenting problem. The derivation of this hypothesis is an integral aspect of the information-gathering assessment and is often referred to as the formulation. The second stage of the assessment demands a more selective collection of data which are used to determine the nature of therapeutic strategies and then assist in monitoring the state of change the clients go through. This style of assessment should be a continuous process as long as the client remains in a therapeutic situation.

Increasingly, however, the distinction between these two styles of assessment is becoming blurred. For example, in forensic psychology, a client could be a child or young person subject to serious injury during a road traffic accident. It would be most unusual for the damages due to that child to be assessed purely on the basis of initial information-gathering conducted on a one-off basis. Although such assessments could occur, the result would lead to recommendations for appropriate therapeutic input (e.g. physiotherapy, occupational therapy, speech therapy) and the outcome of these remedial approaches would be reviewed periodically until such time as it was clear that the client's special needs were resolved or unlikely to alter. Similarly, in the child protection arena an abusive parent may receive an in-depth risk assessment of the information-gathering type and then be subjected to a therapeutic process designed to lessen the risk presented. The rehabilitation of a child to this parent might well be determined by the degree of change evident as a consequence of the therapeutic input. In some cases, the limitations of the information-gathering model lead inevitably to a conclusion that the clinician cannot be certain that the client is capable of change. It may well be recommended that a process of 'therapeutic assessment' be initiated such that the client is subject to therapeutic processes with the goal of assessing whether or not he or she is capable of benefiting from them in the long term and within a time-scale appropriate to the child's changing needs (Fitzpatrick, 1995).

Inevitably the clinician's experience is that clients respond to feedback from assessments, even information-gathering assessments, by making changes. It would appear that participating in the act of assessment draws the attention of the client to salient issues which had not been considered in depth previously. Changes seem to occur particularly when clients are included as participants in the assessment process through the discussion of the reasons for assessment, reflection on the facts given by the clients during the assessment, discussion of test results and their interpretation (e.g. Allen, 1981; Fischer, 1994; Jaffe, 1988). Not surprisingly, such observations have caused clinicians to wonder whether there is any meaningful distinction between assessment and treatment. Thus, Allen (1981) stated that assessment was a 'treatment in microcosm' (p. 251). Despite these blurred distinctions and interlinked situations, the differences between the two styles of assessment are, however, sufficiently robust and important to justify their continued separation.

Contrasting the information-gathering model with the therapeutic model

The two models can be differentiated along a number of dimensions. This differentiation is described briefly in order that the subsequent description of assessment in respect of workplace bullying can be placed most particularly within the information-gathering model.

The distinction between the two has, most recently, been thoroughly identified by Finn and Tonsager (1997). Their analysis begins with an evaluation of the different goals of the two models. They point out that the information-gathering model is used primarily as a means of improving communication with the clients so that decisions can be made about them. The presenting problems of the clients are evaluated and placed within clinical descriptions and categories that are already well researched. Thus, one client who has experienced extreme stress as a result of workplace bullying might show sufficient difficulties to fulfil diagnostic criteria of post-traumatic stress disorder (PTSD) as defined by DSM-IV and/or ICD-10 – these being the two foremost international classifications of mental disorders. Another victim, subject to extreme workplace bullying, may present problems that go beyond PTSD and fulfil the criteria for obsessive-compulsive disorder (OCD).

On the face of it, such attempts to categorise clients may be seen as dehumanising them or removing their individuality. Nevertheless, such descriptions are important; they may help to determine whether the client can work again or be seen as so disabled as to be unable to have employment in any environment. Across the board of psychological assessment, such descriptions are frequently the basis for vital conclusions. A client may have such special needs as to justify primary care management; another may be defined as so risky as to be unable to parent a child; and others are defined as having such levels of adult dependency and other special needs that important services must be provided for them.

Quite clearly such decisions are facilitated by strategies of assessment that have established reliability such that the validity of the conclusions is open to inspection by other psychologists. Such assessments move from the particular case of the individual to the generality of psychological knowledge of his or her presenting problems. If this validity is not apparent then the assessment is without value.

By contrast, the therapeutic model has, as its major goal, the active process of ensuring that the client is provided with new understanding of experiences such that he or she can find avenues for positive change in their life. The clinician's primary objective is not to make judgments on the adequacy or veracity of the client's account but to be attentive to and reflective on those presentations. The goal is to increase opportunities for insight which may leave the client better able to reappraise their situation and so function in more adaptive ways. Finn and Tonsager state: 'In many ways, the goals of therapeutic assessment parallel the aims of all psychotherapies, because all are committed to helping people confirm, challenge, and change how they act, think, and feel about themselves' (1997, p. 378).

Process

The information-gathering model generally relies on a three-step process for complete assessment. The first is essentially one of data collection which will probably be systematised under various headings (see below) including psychometric assessment wherever possible; second is the deductive interpretation of the data gained; and the third concerns the recommendations arising from the clinician's conclusions. Clearly the second stage is that where the clinician endeavours to interpret the data taken to develop understanding of the client. It is not often the case that the client has any part in constructing these interpretations other than that of providing information. In addition, the conclusions and recommendations are made without negotiation with the client, and it is usually only after these are formed that the client is given any feedback. It is good clinical practice for the client to see the report that the clinician produces eventually and to discuss this. Clearly, where legal proceedings are ongoing the client is unlikely to get this report directly but will receive it through his or her solicitors. Often it is the case that the solicitor must discuss this report with a barrister and seek further information from the clinician before the client has a chance of feedback. This process is common in respect of workplace bullying.

Therapeutic assessments proceed in a completely different fashion. The client is much more involved at all levels and, although similar assessment instruments (e.g. interviews, psychometric testing, details from documents) may be used, the client is directly included in the assimilation and interpretation of these. The clinician must work to develop and maintain efficient and empathetic communication with the clients and work collaboratively with the client to formulate the assessment goals. This involves sharing results at all stages and general openness about the clinician's thoughts about the presenting problems.

It can be seen from this description that the clients are much more likely to be collaborative with the therapeutic assessment process in an active way because they are encouraged to participate in all the different aspects of their assessment. Thus, for example, it would not be unusual for a clinician to discuss test results with the client in order to discover how these are viewed compared with the client's self-constructs. Such a partnership is more likely to establish robust strategies for dealing with the presenting problems not only for the present but throughout the rest of the client's life course.

Standardised tests

The purpose of standardised tests is to compare some aspect(s) of the client's behaviour or cognition (attitudes, beliefs, personality mediators) with a normative sample. In doing so, the test results take the direction of the assessment away from the client's interview response and personal history into the larger world of the population from which the normative sample was drawn. Thus, for example, the degree of extroversion shown by an employee in his or her own workplace could be compared with the norm provided by a large sample of employees across workplace environments. In addition, if that employee completes a psychometric schedule on his or her interpersonal behaviour, then the probability of, for example, this person displaying levels of verbal aggression beyond the norm could be determined. It is clear, therefore, that such psychometric instruments enable not only comparison of the client with a norm but also predictions of future levels of behaviour. Psychometric tests are highly valued but only if they are shown to be valid, stable and reliable and have the ability to make accurate predictions. Thus, only those instruments that have a good track record of research and replication studies could fulfil these criteria.

The main difference between the two models of assessment in the usage of such tests is that the therapeutic model makes use of the tests' results to facilitate the client's understanding through decision and explanation. It is much less likely that a clinician working to the information-gathering model would go through such a process with the client, for fear of contaminating other aspects of information-gathering. It is not desirable that clients show significant change during the processes of information-gathering as these changes may be only temporary and render invalid previously gathered information.

The biggest single difference, therefore, between the two models in respect of the use of tests is that the information-gathering model makes use of them mainly from the nomothetic perspective, whereas the therapeutic assessment model takes an ideographic perspective. In many situations, forensic psychological assessments have to be safeguarded against any tendency for the assessor to become too linked empathetically to the client. This difficulty has been referred to as the 'clinical hermeneutics error' (Harkness and Lilienfeld, 1997, p. 350) where the clinician unwittingly becomes trapped in the client's perspective such that underlying psychopathology becomes seen increasingly as normal variation. When this happens in relation to legal proceedings, then, quite correctly, the other parties may claim that the clinician has become too partisan to provide a reliable expert opinion.

The importance of data

As far as the information-gathering model is concerned, data are important only because they enable a variation displayed by the client to be assessed in relation to a normative population. Thus, for example, a victim of workplace bullying may seek damages because he or she has sustained post-traumatic stress disorder but the claim will not be upheld if the assessment does not provide data indicating that the client fulfils the diagnostic criteria of PTSD. The interpersonal link between clinician and client is not ignored within the information-gathering model but is valued solely because it facilitates good communication and increases the probability of accurate data gathering.

Conversely the importance of data to a therapeutic assessment is that they can provide a dynamic rather than static view of the client's adaptive change, such that the eventual outcome of the assessment is less important than the changes promoted by its process. As a consequence, the dynamic relationship between client and clinician is important not only for the acquisition of data but also as a vehicle for promoting change. It is vital that the clinician experiences empathy for the client and respects that in the interpersonal dynamics of the assessment sessions.

As may be seen, the essential differences concerning the importance of data are inextricably linked to differences in the roles of the clinicians using information-gathering or therapeutic assessment models. The information-gathering approach, particularly as it is used in respect of legal proceedings, demands that the clinician retain objectivity of detachment such that the data from which the formulation is distilled are as objectively obtained as possible. The clinician acting in this way is sometimes likened to a scientist examining a sample under a microscope, who functions in such a way that the nature of the sample remains unchanged.

In contrast, however, the clinician who is fulfilling a role within the therapeutic assessment model not only gathers data but seeks to help the client bring about changes which are reflected in significant alterations within data acquired over subsequent sessions. The strong element of subjectivity is encouraged because the client is valued as an individual rather than a member of some normative sample.

The two models can become complementary under certain circumstances. For example, a client who is bedevilled by post-traumatic stress disorder confirmed by a clinician functioning within the information-gathering model may be subjected to a therapeutic assessment by a clinician seeking to determine if change is possible within a reasonable time-scale for the client. It is axiomatic that clients who can demonstrate such changes are less severely damaged than those who cannot, and these differences may be reflected in the quantum of damages.

Information-gathering assessment

The thrust of this book concerns the assessment of victims and perpetrators of workplace bullying. As such, the information-gathering model of assessment is of great significance. This is not to belittle or regard as unimportant the vital role therapeutic assessment has to play in relation to workplace bullying but is a recognition that therapeutic strategies are outside its compass.

There have been many attempts to find the best process for information-gathering assessments (e.g. Nay, 1979; Cone, 1978). The structure presented here is an amalgam and has been found sufficiently robust to 'unpick' the complexities of factors associated with workplace bullying. This framework owes much to the conventional examination of psychiatric patients (e.g. Russell, 1987), augmented by the use of personality assessment tests and other psychological schedules (e.g. Ben-Porath, 1997). As may be seen below, it consists of a number of interlinked stages for gathering data which are brought together into a formulation and then to a set of conclusions. In the context of workplace bullying, these stages can be guided by the model described in Chapter 2.

Identification of client and clinician

This is the preliminary material which identifies the full name, date of birth and address of the client and provides details of the clinician him- or herself. It is customary to add other important details such as the dates over which the assessment occurred and the date upon which the final report was written.

Reports for legal proceedings will also require the professional qualifications of the clinician and a statement of the clinician's expertise, indicating why it is that the clinician is an appropriate person to receive instructions in the matter.

Reason for referral

It is vital that all assessments have clear goals. These may take the form of instructions from a solicitor or result from a clinical team meeting or other source able to provide such instructions. Ideally the client should be aware of these instructions and be familiar with their purpose.

Summary

It is customary for many clinicians, the writer included, to provide a summary at this point stating how the assessment was carried out and what the conclusions were. The purpose of this is to enable readers, particularly those who sent the instructions for the assessment, to learn immediately the outcomes without having to go through all the detail.

Basis of the assessment

This is an important section because it details the sources from which information was gathered and provides an opportunity for the clinician to indicate where, if any, there were gaps. Where the assessment is part of legal proceedings the clinician will invariably have been sent certain documents which provide background material. These documents should provide details of the alleged incidents of bullying but may also contain medical records, employment records, details of the employer's organisation and statements taken from various relevant individuals. The latter might include a statement or statements from the client, witnesses, trade union representatives and medical reports. It is important that all of these are listed so that information gathered from documents is properly identified and can be checked.

This section would also list with dates all interview sessions with the client, psychological testing sessions, discussions with other people, observations of functioning which may have been made, and related telephone conversations with other people who know the difficulties experienced by the client well. These may include parents, spouse, therapists, care staff, social workers, psychologists, general practitioners, etc. Many distressed clients find it difficult to describe their problems successfully and rely heavily upon people close to them to provide detailed information. Where those 'relevant others' are used, their input to the assessment must be carefully noted. It should be stated clearly that the client had given permission for them to be approached.

Documentary information

An integral part of the assessment is a thorough review of whatever documents have been provided about the presenting problem. These should be reviewed carefully and detailed in this section. Where, for example, the client is a victim or an alleged victim of workplace bullying, then the documents should be examined for factors that relate particularly to what is known of workplace bullying. This would include personal details about the client which may be associated, including common 'triggers' such as physical abnormality, wearing of glasses, accent, demeanour, personality traits, etc. Details of the client's employment history may also be provided in the documents and may also be considered relevant. The nature of the client's occupation within the organisation is most likely to be important and this may involve reviewing any documents that deal with the processes by which the client came to have that occupation.

The documents may also give indications of the employment conditions and the 'culture' prevailing in the workplace; these should be considered in detail if possible. It is most important that any statements provided by the client should be cross-referenced to material within the documents if they exist. For example, if a victim of workplace bullying asserts that he or she had endeavoured to engage higher management to stop the problem, then it is helpful to make reference to any letters or memos which support this assertion. Given the material in the preceding chapter which describes why the victims of workplace bullying should be seen to have tried to work within the employment policies of the employer, it is obviously important that the presence or absence of supporting documents should be commented upon.

Likewise, if the client is asserting that they have been so stressed by the incidents of bullying that they became unwell and unable to work, then it is obviously important that the background section deals with any medical documents that support this. Reference to the symptoms of stress, as recorded by general practitioners or psychiatrists, constitutes vital information in the identification of bullying-related symptoms.

On occasions, the documents might also contain comments from observers of the client functioning in the workplace setting which may indicate that the client behaved in such a way as to attract negative evaluations and aggressive responses. It is very important that these documented comments are dealt with and related to the client's perceptions. Dispute-related bullying (see Chapter 1) is no more acceptable than the bullying of a randomly selected target, but the characteristics and behaviour of a client who is perceived to have been provocative may obviously be used in mitigation, and the assessment must deal from the outset with these behaviours and characteristics – otherwise the clinician may be accused of dealing selectively with information.

Particular areas of concern revealed by this review of documentation should be clearly identified and should be seen to be dealt with in the subsequent section which reports on interview sessions with the client.

Interviews with the client

Interview assessments in the area of workplace bullying are no different from other areas where interviews are needed, in that it is important for the clinician to be sharply focused on what information is required, even though in 'telling the story' the client may be allowed as much flexibility as he or she needs to be comfortable. Bearing in mind that interviews are often best seen as conversations with a purpose, it is wise for clinicians not to overly constrain the client by insisting on a rigid format. Distressed or indignant clients may well tend to treat the interview sessions as a cathartic opportunity and so are unlikely to make the clinician's job easier by staying tightly within the frames of reference provided by the clinician's questions. The victims of workplace bullying often retain their sense of shock, shame, embarrassment and indignation for months or years after the events. Post-traumatic stress delays the recovery period and is likely to damage the selective attention of the clients; this is a significant symptom in its own right and should be commented upon. Careful notes are needed so that the clinician can extract relevant information and assign it to appropriate categories after each interview session. It is important not to antagonise distressed clients by over-exhaustive questioning as this may reinforce sad feelings which people do not want to re-experience – they may simply want to get a job of information gathering done as quickly as possible. Similarly, redundant issues should be avoided unless they are needed to help improve responsiveness.

It is often desirable to start reporting the interview sessions by commenting on the **circumstances of the interviews**. This describes briefly where the interviews took place and what the conditions were like. It may also comment on the client's immediate presentation and how this changed (e.g. more to less stressed) as the client became more familiar with the process. Any description of the assessment or its instructions provided to the client should be noted here, along with the comments that have been made in response to this.

Perception of current circumstances

This section reports on the client's description of how they are functioning given that the problems have occurred. It is generally desirable to comment on the current employment status, health and general functioning of the clients giving details of **impairments** which the client associates with the difficulties they have experienced. These often include a worsening of family relationships, loss of colleagues at work, inability to concentrate, inability to enjoy activities of previous interest, difficulties in functioning as a spouse or parent, and general loss of ability to plan and organise daily life routines.

Impairments may also be evident in biological functioning such as sleep patterns, eating disorders and the maintenance of body weight, sexual activity and exercise tolerance. Associated difficulties arising from, for example, poor decision making, inability to manage household budgets, communicating with others, and the effects of stress avoidance strategies should also be described here. Any coping strategies adopted by the client should also be noted. Some may be obviously maladaptive, such as over-consumption of alcohol, taking tranquillisers, much-increased smoking, self-inflicted isolation, excessive dependency, attention seeking and denial. Where such maladaptive strategies exist, it is desirable to gain information about how others, close to the client, are coping. Adaptive coping strategies are also worthy of detail. These might include undertaking assertiveness training, retraining for employment, improving physical fitness and getting engaged in hobbies and interests. Some strategies may appear to be adaptive, such as getting involved in voluntary work, but may be motivated by a morbid need to locate others with worse problems. The prevailing mood of the client is also of great significance and extreme mood variations should be commented upon.

Finally, it is helpful to make a comparison, if possible, between the client's functioning at the time of the assessment and how his or her peers are functioning. Specifically, the question is asked: 'How is this client faring in relation to others who are comparable with him or her in relation to age, gender, qualifications, training, experience, culture and ethnicity?' Any detriments in the comparison could be related to the experience of workplace bullying.

The **personal history** of the client should be taken carefully. This should include an examination of medical and developmental factors of relevance, particularly where, for example, birth injuries may have contributed to deformities or actual handicaps which mark out the individual as different. Educational history is as important, not only in relation to academic achievement and any special educational needs which might still have relevance, but also in respect of the development of peer relations. As stated previously, there is increasing evidence that the victims of workplace bullying may have had experiences of being bullied in childhood at school or in their community and similarly, the perpetrators of workplace bullying are sometimes found to have been the victims of childhood abuse or excessively power-assertive strategies for discipline (Randall, 1997b).

Employment history should be examined with the client, with consideration again of peer relations and prior experience of any abuses in the workplace.

It is tragic that several clinical narrative studies of female workplace victims reveal that they have also experienced domestic violence and become subjugated both at home and the workplace. Obviously where an individual is subjected to stress from more than one environment, then it will be difficult to partial out the effects of one source of stress from another. Perhaps in recognition of that, some victims of workplace bullying are loath to give details of their domestic lives, and several sessions may be required before the client has sufficient confidence to describe the true situation.

The client's description of their workplace experiences has to be carefully cross-referenced to any statement they have produced. Anomalies need to be ironed out such that a full history is obtained, inclusive of the earliest recognised start date, incident-by-incident description, details of observers and of the efforts made to seek change. As far as victims are concerned, it is vitally important that they have attempted to draw their plight to the attention of the employer, making use of whatever appropriate personal harassment policies the employer may have. In those cases where there is no such policy, then the victim should have sought assistance from his or her line manager and, we hope, recorded the outcome.

Given that many victims of workplace bullying take out their frustrations on their employer rather than the perpetrators, it is desirable to ask if the victim felt able to reduce the stress by, perhaps, reducing work output quality or rate, or striking a covert blow in some other way. Such endeavours are particularly common where the perpetrator is the line manager or higher. Workplace victims may be reluctant to give such details because they fear damaging their own case where litigation may be involved. It is, however, desirable that they are honest about such strategies because it is very likely that the employment records will show the impact on their performance.

Other aspects of the interview sessions should cover the client's perception of the workplace environment; whether they have found it to be conducive and relaxed or stressed or threatening. Their comments should relate to what is known about the manifestations of workplace bullying in different employment cultures in order to facilitate those aspects of the formulation that deal with the particular client experience of bullying within his or her particular workplace environment.

When rounding up the sessions, the clinician may become interested again in the client's mood states and wish to record evidence of fear, frustration, anger, sadness, anxiety and irritation or evidence of flatness of affect. Absence of variation in facial expression should not be taken to indicate that the client is emotionless (Ekman and Oster, 1979), but further information on the client's emotional state may need to be sought from relevant others such as spouse or parents.

Both victims and perpetrators of workplace bullying may experience some thought disorder. This is not uncommon and more often than not is stress-related. This is troublesome. Preoccupations or intrusive thoughts may characterise times of particular stress or distress, and there may also be evidence of abnormal beliefs about the environment and those people who share it with the client. Low self-esteem, chronic negative self-evaluation and feelings of unworthiness are common amongst workplace victims whereas perpetrators may overestimate their abilities and value to the organisation. There may also be differentiation over perception of control; workplace victims, may feel completely vulnerable and totally exposed to factors outside of themselves, whereas perpetrators may exude confidence and a belief that they are fully in control of their lives. The interview session may also give evidence of severe thought disorder and abnormal experiences along the auditory, visual or other sensory modalities. Clients experiencing severe stress may report hallucinations or strong feelings of being unreal. Semantic sensations such as numbness in fingers and toes may be reported along with psychotic episodes of disturbed thinking. Paranoid thinking is commonly found during assessments relating to workplace bullying and need not be indicative of a severe mental health disorder.

Impaired intellectual functioning may be evident during the interview session in terms of memory dysfunction, disorientation in time or space, attention deficit and an inability to concentrate. Such difficulties may have a significant impact on an employee functioning at work and lead to critical and/or aggressive behaviour interpreted as bullying. Such descriptions would have to be assessed and this provides an obvious role for psychometric evaluation. Cognitive dysfunction may be evident also in the attitudes the client has towards his or her life. Some clients may have a hopelessly idealistic vision of returning to work, renewed, well-supported and able to progress as never before. Other clients may view their situation as hopeless and perceive them-selves as condemned to a life marred by stress, inability to relate to people, constant suspicion and avoidance. Examination of the client's medical history is particularly important to determine if there have been any previous psychological and psychiatric problems, and what, if any, treatment has been received for them. The role of medication should be investigated at this point, particularly if there are side-effects that could affect the client's judgement in complex social situations such as the workplace environment.

Psychometric testing

The information thus gathered from the preceding stages would provide indications of areas for assessment through psychometric testing. For example, the presentation of the client might be indicative of learning difficulty, in which case intellectual testing might be required. Failure to demonstrate episodic memory in relation to relating his or her history might suggest that some form of memory assessment would be appropriate.

Comparatively brief assessments of intellectual capability could be made by using relatively simple format tests such as the Ravens Progressive Matrices and the Mill Hill Vocabulary test. Although quite aged these tests do have good reliability and validity; they are sufficiently robust to provide indications for further testing if necessary.

The Weschler Adult Intelligence Scale in its most recent revised version (WAIS-III) is the most popular test available for sensitive determination of cognitive abilities, strengths and weaknesses. The Weschler Memory Scales have the same statistical basis as the WAIS-III and enable comprehensive assessment of memory dysfunction which may be a symptom of post-traumatic stress.

The most frequent psychometric assessments are those associated with personality and personal-social functioning. Measurements of stress levels associated with the effects of workplace bullying are needed frequently and other measures used might tap self-esteem and interpersonal behaviour. It is often useful to investigate the client's social network independently of their own information. Lack of social support contributes to the level of distress experienced by people and is likely to increase dependency on professional agencies.

Suitable tests for these aspects of the assessment are described in the next chapter.

Formulation

This part of the assessment examines the psychological knowledge base that relates to the presenting problems of the client in respect of workplace bullying. The formulation should consider what is known of antecedent consequences and liken this to the difficulty experienced by the client. The possible outcomes, in terms of severity, should be considered within the framework of the legal context of bullying. The guidance provided by the Judicial Studies Board (2000) is invaluable.

Wherever possible it is desirable to demonstrate what effort should be made by employers to prevent workplace bullying, in order to present a basis for the opinions and conclusions which are stated subsequently.

Opinions and conclusions

The opinions section examines the information gathered alongside the relevant research and psychological knowledge base to provide objective answers to the questions of the instructions. The stated opinions should make clear how they are derived and not provide any new information or research material not already debated. Any conclusions drawn and recommendations from them should be stated separately and quoted in the summary section early on in the report.

Examples of reports using this structure are provided in the last chapter.

Clinical narrative as a tool of assessment

As indicated above, no assessment of victims or bullies can be complete without a detailed case history. Such histories are constructed out of narrative structures provided by the person being assessed, and used by the clinician to assist in developing the formulation. Such use of narrative is accepted as vital to the investigation process, yet, increasingly, similar approaches to psychology, psychiatry and psychotherapy have progressively attached less importance to this type of investigation at the nomothetic level.

Many exponents of the use of clinical narrative complain that the modern-day process of completing case histories is dehumanising because the subjective experiences of the person are made impersonal (e.g. Hauerwas, 1993). Crossley (2000) describes how social constructionist approaches have begun to replace humanistic interpretations of an individual's narrative by emphasising linguistic and cultural structures over the individual's concept of 'self'. Although there are several different social constructionist approaches, a common theme is that 'self' does not exist independently of the changing experiences of daily living and the way that individuals use language to interpret and account for their actions in respect of them. In brief, the deconstruction of 'self' is an inevitable consequence of this constant renewal process. In turn, this begs the question as to whether the case history approach to assessment can ever reveal some essential nature of the client which is independent of what happens to him or her. In the context of workplace bullying, this view could assert that findings concerning the personalities of victims are simply descriptions of the results of bullying

rather than of pre-bullying traits leading to targeting by bullies. Social facilitation and impression management effects may be active also such that the
victims are likely to create a perspective of 'self' that is essentially innocent
within the relationship they have with their bullies.

This viewpoint has many advocates. For example, Cox and Theilgaard
(1987) state that the way in which individuals see the world is only from
their own perspective; this is unlikely to be objective or historically accurate.
The accounts given about important life events are inevitably tainted by
differing perspectives at different stages of life and by a desire to provoke or
evoke different responses from different listeners. Frank (1993) is robust in
stating that life stories are both highly selected and selective accounts. The
individual is seen not so much as remembering history but reconstructing
it from the accretion of evidence, moulding it to suit the occasion and
the desired response from the listener. It is not surprising, therefore, that
Peneff (1990, ch. 1) notes that most life stories contain few immoral or
otherwise undesirable acts. By the same token many life stories are not
reflexive; there is little pondering or reinterpretation that weakens the
perspective individuals use to account for themselves or their actions. The
process of taking a case history can readily provide an opportunity for
the enhancement of self-image.

Yet this apparent omission of reflexivity by the social constructionist
approaches flies in the face of everyday human behaviour as it is observed.
Parker (1991) argues that this capacity is central to the concept of personal
agency which mediates social behaviour. Even at the basic level of 'If I do
that, this person may not like me', it is obvious that reflexivity functions as a
consistent trait of individuals to assist them to operate in their social world. It
is, perhaps, the process of discourse in providing the life history that leads to
the unrealistic representation of 'self'. The alternative is that people do not
process any fundamental sense of their own 'self' and cannot function as
purposeful agents in shaping their lives from the events around them.
Augustinous and Walker (1995) point to the inevitable conclusion drawn
from this viewpoint that 'there is little beyond a personal psychology which is
a moment-to-moment situated experience' (p. 276).

Attempts made to incorporate a sense of personal agency and reflexivity
include the Interpretative Phenomenological Analysis described by Smith
(1996). He and his colleagues are concerned with subjectivity in terms of how
people think and feel about what happens to them. Their subjectivities are
presumed to be connected to themselves and events by a domain of facts that
may be uncovered and investigated using particular approaches. Narrative
psychology is believed to be an appropriate strategy and one that enables
investigation of a person's sense of 'self' which transcends daily experiences.
Crossley states that theories of narrative psychology allow the argument
that 'human life carries within it a narrative structure to the extent that the
individual, at the level of trait, phenomenological experience, is constantly

projecting backwards and forwards in a manner that maintains a sense of coherence, unity, meaningfulness and identity' (Crossley, 2000, p. 542).

Traumatic events may disrupt this process seriously and Crossley illustrates this by considering the impact of experiencing serious illness. She states that the disruption caused by trauma interrupts the maintenance of coherence and identity in time, space and person, which would be recognisable to clinicians making a mental state examination. By the same token, the gradual reintroduction of the narrative structure can assist the individual to recover their sense of identity and re-establish a new pattern of adaptive functioning.

It is from this basis that the author believes that the narratives provided by clients not only display the damage done to them by the traumatic experiences of adult bullying but also reveal their symbolisation of 'self' which they endeavour to re-connect during recovery. In this way one can give credence to their depiction of pre-trauma functioning, belief, attitudes and traits.

Part 2

Characteristics of perpetrators

Chapter 4

Bully characteristics: personal history and development

It is a sad fact that some small children carry with them characteristics, sometimes indefinable, which cause experienced teachers and social workers to predict that they will become aggressive perpetrators who are likely to cause harm to their peers or others in some way. This early damning of a child may be unprofessional, discriminatory and set to create a self-fulfilling prophecy but still it happens because many of the predictions are accurate. Some children do grow up to follow in the troubled footsteps of their parents or older siblings; their disaffection and hostility evident at school perhaps turns to delinquency and violence when out of it. This cycle of hostility and aggression is clearly evident when young people turn to lawbreaking in the same way as their older siblings or parents; different professionals will see the same cyclic phenomena operating within the school, the home and the community (Randall, 1996).

Lay people recognise the process also; they state 'There is no wonder he's a bully, look at the home he comes from.' They, like the teachers and social workers, are aware that aggressive children are often the products of aggressive parenting and other faulty socialisation processes. Their general perspective is that aggression is often learned during the developmental processes of childhood and there is good evidence to support them (e.g. Tremblay, 2000). Most people understand that no child comes into the world with a gene for bullying biding its time for the right environment in which to flourish; instead they understand that bullies are the product of complex social processes which, through faulty learning, create an antisocial personality characterised by the aggressive manipulation of other people. Unless their poor socialisation is repaired during childhood, it is likely that these children will become the perpetrators of workplace bullying, domestic violence and other hostile behaviours.

This sad process makes school-based interventions very important; not only may they enable prospective victims of school bullying to study and develop in peace and security, but also spare the workplace of later problems as well. Fortunately, school-based interventions are effective. Thus Olweus (1993) was able to demonstrate a 50 per cent reduction in school bullying after two years of the Norwegian programme, and Smith and Sharp (1994) reported reductions of between 15 and 20 per cent in the UK. Other studies have reported moderate reductions in Canada (Pepler, Craig, Zeigler and Charach, 1993) and the UK (Pitts and Smith, 1994).

No matter how good the interventions may be, not all school bullying is vanquished; a hard core of bullies remain impervious (Smith and Sharp, 1994) and some may even be stimulated to bully in association with the interventions (Randall, 1996). The students enjoy the bullying and gain significant reinforcement from it (Randall, 1997). Others become both irritant and bully, the 'provocative victims' best described by Pikas (1989), and so invite bullying, whilst others become both bully and victim (Bowers, Smith and Binney, 1994), with very complex needs outside the influence of school intervention programmes. Clinical investigation of these students reveals that most have significant difficulties within the context of their home life, and family-based interventions are needed (Randall, 1996; Smith and Myron-Wilson, 1998).

This chapter examines some of the processes associated with parenting style, attachment and socialisation which contribute to the derivation of the bully personality profile.

Aggression and the preschool period

It is a mistake to believe that young children are unable to develop a propensity for bullying. Recent research suggests that the behaviour may become evident from the age of 4 years (Szegal, 1985). Diagnostic work with preschool children reveals a collection of antisocial behavioural symptoms which include extreme aggressiveness with tantrums, gross stubbornness with severe noncompliance, very poor responses to limits and rules, and generally poor control and expression of emotions (e.g. Campbell, 1990).

Child development, aggression and its inhibitions

The propensity to aggression forms part of normal development (Parke and Slaby, 1983), but it is also the case that the acquisition of inhibitory controls is also a part of the same developmental process. As aggression develops through its various stages (Szegal, 1985), so inhibitions grow to mediate the production of aggressive behaviour (Cicchetti, Ganiban and Barnett, 1990). In this way aggressive tendencies are prevented from developing unchecked in most children.

During the first stage to 12 months, the development of early forms of aggression and the growing ability of infants to regulate it may be observed. Angry behaviour can be provoked in neonates (e.g. Campos, Barrett, Lamb, Goldsmith and Steinberg, 1983) but the soothing response of the parents helps the infant to stabilise. Early expressions of anger can evolve into intentionally aggressive behaviour when representations of self, object and goal-seeking behaviours co-exist (Edgecumbe and Sandler, 1974). Most researchers (e.g. Harding, 1983; Kagan, 1974) believe that the age at which this develops is somewhere between 4 and 10 months. It is likely, therefore, that infants develop rudimentary aggressive intentional behaviour during that period.

Szegal's observational studies indicate that the first clear evidence of intentional aggression occurs between 7 and 12 months as a response typically to painful stimuli or discomfort, experiences of tension or frustration, and at times when the infant demands attention. Others (e.g. Parens, 1979) believe, however, that this intentional behaviour occurs earlier, perhaps as young as 5 months, as infants develop an awareness of separateness from their primary caregivers.

Mediation of aggression begins during the first year as part of the development of a wide range of affect regulation skills. These enable the infant to redirect, control, change and bring about adaptive functioning in emotionally arousing situations (Cicchetti, Ganiban and Barnett, 1990). Later, children develop the skills for behaving acceptably even in situations that are tense, emotional and frequent antecedents to aggression or other undesirable behaviours.

From 3 months to the end of the first year the infant's capacity and desire for social interaction grow significantly. Parallel with this comes the satisfaction of increasing skill in producing effects on the environment (e.g. banging pram rattles, holding objects). These interactions enable infants to be less dependent on adults for stimulation and so they become less susceptible (e.g. Burns, 1986) to frustration. By 12 months another critical development has usually occurred. Infants start to organise cognitive and behavioural expressions in respect of their primary caregivers, usually the mother. The combination of these factors may be understood as an attachment relationship which comes to fulfil an increasingly complex and valuable function for the developing child. Main, Kaplan and Cassidy (1985) stated that the quality of interactions with the principal carer is of critical importance during this period and the satisfaction derived by the infants does much to increase the rate at which aggression becomes controllable. The infant is therefore more able to tolerate tensions and stresses without the need to respond aggressively.

Aggressive behaviour shows a significant increase in frequency from about 18 months to 2 years. Szegal (1985) suggests that children are so used to all their needs being met instantly that they cannot accept anything less from their carers. Parens (1979) believes that they do not associate immediately the carers who force deferment of gratification and frustration with those who are also their main sources of pleasure and need gratification. That this inability to recognise the carers in both roles, and so 'forgive' delays imposed by them, leads to aggression which continues into the third year of life and which is at the root of the characteristic temper tantrums of the 'terrible twos'. Other researchers (e.g. Mahler, Pine and Bergman, 1975) believe that this increase of aggression is also a result of the children's desire to develop increasing autonomy by using aggressive behaviour.

The desire to acquire objects such as toys becomes associated frequently with instances of aggressive behaviour in nursery settings (e.g. Szegal, 1985). Later difficulties with peer relations appear to have their roots in behaviour of this sort, and most children are capable of showing a full range of negative, as well as positive, emotions by their third birthday. This includes obvious emotions such as anger caused by jealousy and also subtle emotional expressions as well. For example, Dunn (1992) has shown that the subtle range enables children as young as 18 months to premeditate getting their siblings into trouble.

The most important source of affect regulation at this age arises with the development of representation through language and symbolic play (Main *et al.* 1985). Representation is vital for the development of the modification and control of behaviour associated with emotional expression during this period (Emde, 1985). As language becomes more elaborate and useful to the child, so it is used increasingly to reduce frustration and anxiety throughout the second and third years. Children become able to use simple negotiation strategies based on expressive language instead of coercive strategies based on aggression (Cicchetti, Cummings, Greenberg and Marvin, 1990).

Another important regulator of aggression is the children's increasing ability to cope with the inhibition of their behaviour caused by 'rules' set by adults. Children as young as 18 months can modify their behaviour according to limits even when the primary rule-maker is not present (Vaughn, Kopp and Kurakow, 1984). This suggests that they are able to 'internalise' simple rules and not rely on the antecedents supplied by the presence of the principal rule-makers. Similarly, Power and Chapieski (1986) found that 2-year-olds were capable of maintaining rule-prescribed behaviour even when their primary carers were not present.

The ability to follow rules is a part of the increasing social awareness of the young child and is also associated with the development of an empathetic response to the distress of others. Some authors (e.g. Eisenberg and Mussen, 1989) have described a sympathetic behavioural response from children as young as 18 months. This development is associated with early pro-social behaviour and indicates that children now realise that they live in a world inhabited by others who also have feelings. Empathy is, of course, an important inhibitor of aggressive behaviour. This development implies also that 'theory of mind' is being acquired in that the children are able to understand that others are having feelings independently of themselves. It has been suggested that bullies who seem genuinely unable to understand the depth of hurt that they cause may be deficient in the development of theory of mind (Randall, 1998).

The development between 2 and 3 years is characterised by a marked increase in the rate of aggression, and also the nature of the aggression changes markedly. The increase continues until about two and a half years and then gradually reverses. More importantly, verbal aggression expands in type and content as behaviours such as biting, hair-pulling, deliberately aiming and throwing objects, hitting, kicking and pushing show reduction (Cicchetti, Cummings, *et al.* 1990; Stern, 1985). Several researchers have shown that children as young as two and a half years of age can express their aggression verbally and also begin to justify it in a rudimentary way (e.g. Miller and Sperry, 1987). Much of this verbal aggression is associated with compliance refusal. Unfortunately the welcome change from physical to verbal aggression is somewhat mitigated by the fact that instances of physical aggression last longer than they used to (Fagot and Hagan, 1985).

The regulation of aggressive behaviour also improves during this period. Language and the ability to play alongside other children without territorial incidents have become much more refined and opportunities for hostility and danger are thereby diminished. Well-regulated children are now able to talk about their feelings and this in turn facilitates their control over the non-verbal expression of strong emotions (Bretherton, Fritz, Zahn-Waxler and Ridgeway, 1986). The period between 3 and 5 years shows a continued marked increase in the amount of time children spend in social interactions without physical fighting. Anger is expressed but it is usually done so verbally or with the use of demonstrative body language. Such 'squabbles' generally occur over possession (Ramsey, 1987). Also at this time children start the complex process of internalising the rules and standards given to them by their parents, older siblings and teachers, and they identify with the people who have provided those rules and standards. The modelling of social behaviour by the child's carers is very important during this time, and with it comes the slow development of conscience that enables children to delay the gratification of impulses (Freud, 1968). This frees them from reliance on controls provided by others and other forms of control that are external to them. Their capacity for empathy develops and gradually they are able to accept that other people have a perspective that is different from their own (e.g. Marcus, Roke and Bruner, 1985). As Campbell (1990) states, they develop a sense of personal responsibility which goes along with a desire to please. These factors, combined also with an urge to succeed, become the tools for successful early social adjustment at school and the foundations for satisfactory academic achievement.

Aggression and assertion

As is evident from the material given above, the inhibition of aggression and the development of pro-social behaviour are dependent upon a successful combination of biological maturation and the adequacy of the environment as contributed mainly by the child's parents or primary caregivers. It is upon these that the complex development of vital component traits such as empathy and self-inhibition is particularly dependent (Kopp, 1982). There are increasing trends away from this form of socialisation as some community investigations (Randall and Donohue, 1993) and nursery school observational studies (e.g. McQuire and Richman, 1986) show that the numbers of aggressive preschool children are growing. Many of these children develop behaviour disorders (Landy and Peters, 1992) and seem not to be receiving, despite adequate biological maturation, the kind of interactions they need from their primary carers which encourage the inhibition of later aggression (Randall, 1993). Indeed, Pettit, Harrist, Bates and Dodge (1991) reported that aggressiveness in kindergarten children is related to a high level of coercive and intrusive family interactions.

In part this may be due to the fact that parents confuse aggression with assertion and believe that the complexities and stressors of modern society require children to be aggressive. They are unaware that aggressive and assertive behaviours are independent categories of response. From as far back as the early 1970s, it was recognised that even so-called 'assertiveness trainers' failed to draw the distinction. Thus Lazarus (1973) stated, 'There is little to be gained, (and much to be lost) from the acquisition of abrasive and obnoxious behaviours in the guise of "assertiveness training"' (p. 698).

Assertiveness has been conceptualised as 'behaviour directed toward reaching some desired goal which continues in the direction of that goal in spite of obstacles in the environment or the opposition of others' (Mauger and Adkinson, 1980, p.1). The attitude of assertive people towards others is generally held to be positive and action taken to secure goals is not aimed primarily at the attacking of obstructive individuals. Violence is used only as self-defence and rules are obeyed in competitions.

Aggressive behaviour, however, emanates from hostile attitudes and its primary purpose is to attack other individuals or exert power over them. The rights of others are disregarded and/or violated. Competitions are marred by aggressive rule-breaking such as deliberately fouling an opponent.

As assertive behaviours may occasionally look very aggressive, the distinction between assertive and aggressive individuals is made according to the intentions of the individuals concerned. The socialisation of individuals depends for its success on the inculcation of socially acceptable attitudes, which allow assertive behaviours but not aggressive ones. Indeed, as all parents know, the socialisation of children is a fraught and complex process if aggression is to be properly channelled into assertiveness, and hostility is to be shaped into pro-social attitudes. These are reviewed here.

From birth, the quality of the contacts between the primary caregiver, usually the mother, and the infant is critical because these should provide a sensitive response to the infant's needs. If these contacts are satisfying then physiological regulation will be established for the infant. In addition, the patterns of interaction begin to be formed which later become the basis for social relationships and styles of interacting with other people (Tronick, 1989); for example, a happy emotional tone based on loving affection during early and subsequent contacts between infants, young children and their caregivers is shown to be crucial for emotional development and the regulation of behaviour (Tronick, 1989). Not surprisingly, Mackinnonlewis, Lamb, Arbuckle, Baradaran and Volling (1992) demonstrated that the most aggressive sons and mothers were dyads who perceived hostile intent in the other; and the efficacy of social adjustment in middle childhood is known to be highly dependent upon the security of preschool attachments (Booth, Rose-Krasnor, McKinnon and Rubin, 1994).

Not only do infants and young children mirror their caregiver's emotional behaviour, they are guided also by facial and vocal displays during emotional expression. Their understanding of the effective products of emotional behaviours follows soon and is used to structure subsequent behaviour. Parents who use pleasing, happy and calming interactions are more likely to modify negative emotional states to more positive ones, especially when anger, sadness and frustration threaten to overwhelm their infants (Klinnert, Campos, Sorce, Emde and Svejda, 1983).

The interactions of the parents and others (e.g. childminders) are vital from another viewpoint. Children are helped to become more able to tolerate frustrating events because of the quality of these interactions and, more specifically, are helped to use language and play to offset much aggressive behaviour linked to frustration. Successful parents 'allow' their children to be angry and to show strong emotions but also encourage them to use speech to represent feelings. This helps the children to 'label' their feelings and so reduce the need to use more physical forms of aggression.

It is known that the behaviour of primary carers becomes a model for the child's subsequent behaviour (e.g. Bandura, Ross and Ross, 1961). Just as carers could model aggression, so they could also model empathy, negotiation, turn taking, caring, comforting and other pro-social behaviours. This modelling, combined with the children's growing capacity for empathy, ensures that, over time, they are more likely to inhibit aggressive behaviour in order to avoid causing pain to other people.

Successful parents provide appropriate limits for behaviour (e.g. Herbert, 1985) and gain attention to these by using successful behaviour management techniques. Typically positive pro-social behaviours are reinforced and aggressive or other undesirable behaviours are sanctioned. Once parents have evolved successful strategies of this sort, they are likely to use them consistently and the children become able, eventually, to internalise the limits that are set. Often the first overt sign that this has not happened properly is when a child's behaviour is found to be difficult and hard to control at school. Investigation of these children frequently reveals the damaged attachments arising from very poor parenting styles (e.g. Smith and Myron-Wilson, 1998).

Parenting style as a function of attitude

Clinical narrative studies of the author suggest that the parents of bullies recognise that their children were angry and hard to handle from the pre-school years. The evolution into bullying often comes as no surprise but they do wonder why and question what went wrong. One explanation is that infant aggression persists because of insecure attachment to the parents, particularly the mother. This argument has its roots in attachment theory and the consequences of parental behaviour during the infancy of their child (e.g. Greenberg and Speltz, 1988). Attachment researchers (e.g. Erickson, Sroufe and Egeland, 1985) point to the withdrawn, angry and often explosive behaviour shown by infants whose parents are distant, reactive and inconsistent. Several studies have linked features of insecure attachment during infancy and early childhood to later difficulties of peer relations, including unpopularity, poor socialisation, elevated aggression with peers and difficulties with affect regulation and conflict resolution (e.g. Matas, Arend and Sroufe, 1978; Cohn, 1990; Booth, Rose-Krasnor and Rubin, 1991).

The data obtained by many research studies, however, have not given firm support to a simple link between insecure attachments and later aggressive behaviour (e.g. Erickson *et al*. 1985). Whereas insecurity may be a factor influencing aggressive behaviour during the preschool years, it appears to act as an antecedent *only* if there is ongoing family stress. Lyons-Ruth, Alpern and Repacholi (1993) studied a carefully selected high-risk, multi-problem sample and reported that a combination of maternal psychological problems and poor attachment predicted higher probability of aggressive behaviour in preschool.

CASE STUDY

Kerry had struggled all through her primary school years with persistent traits of aggression, bullying and peer rivalry. By the age of 13 she was permanently excluded from school because of the escalation of her bullying. Three weeks after the exclusion she was deemed to be out of her mother's control and was removed into local authority care.

This was not a sudden, overnight decision; social workers had had concerns about Kerry and her single-parent mother for periods throughout eleven years. The latter had had periods of amphetamine abuse and on two occasions had been hospitalised. She experienced severe paranoid episodes as a result of her drug habit and was in hospital once for ten weeks to help her overcome a particularly severe psychotic episode induced by the drug. Kerry had been 11 years old at that time and was taken into short-term foster care.

Kerry developed a reputation for persistent bullying from the nursery, aged 4 years. These problems abated at times but at others, usually associated with stress at home, they became intense and temporary exclusions were thought necessary. On one occasion she spoke to a social worker and likened her behaviour at school to the behaviour of her mother; 'She was always scrapping and getting away with it so I thought that was what I should do.'

The mothers of aggressive children hold beliefs about social development that are significantly at variance from those of mothers whose children demonstrate normal social behaviours (Rubin and Mills, 1992). This finding is independent of socio-economic status. The effect is evident when the mothers teach their children about friendship and sharing; the mothers of aggressive preschool children are more likely to believe that their children need to learn these skills through highly direct teaching. They are less skilled than the mothers of non-aggressive children in enabling their children to learn through experimentation and they deny opportunities to consider alternative perspectives. In addition, these mothers block the consequences of various styles of interactive behaviour for themselves and for their children. In general these mothers tell their children how to behave and expect that this will be a sufficient lesson (Sigel, 1982). Their strategies have been referred to as 'low distancing' teaching styles and are associated with later poor performance in the development of interpersonal problem-solving skills (McGulliciddy-deLisi, 1982).

Gardner (1989) matched children rated as aggressive and difficult to manage by their parents and preschool teachers with controls who showed acceptable behaviour. Detailed observations carried out in the home showed that not only were the subject group more likely to refuse maternal instructions but also that their mothers were likely to engage in confrontational behaviour and directive management with their children. Also these mothers were less likely than the mothers of the control group to follow through to compliance. This suggests that the children subjected to directive teaching are less likely to learn compliance and their mothers are less likely to persist. The children are therefore subject to inconsistency; on the one hand these mothers are being directive, but on the other hand they let the children off readily in comparison to the mothers of non-aggressive children (Rubin and Mills, 1992).

One possible explanation given for the contrast is that the mothers of the aggressive children are themselves intimidated by the aggressive behaviour. In an attempt to deal with the tension this causes they may be tempted to believe that it is merely the product of a short-lived phase and so use non-confrontational strategies in order to keep the peace (Patterson, 1982, 1986). Inconsistent styles of management are inevitable and this is known to perpetuate high levels of aggression (Gibb and Randall, 1989). Sadly, the mothers of aggressive children frequently do not see themselves as having any responsibility for the development of this behaviour. Instead they are more likely to attribute it to internal or temperamental factors (Rubin, Mills and Rose-Krasnor, 1989) or external biochemical influences such as food additives (Gibb and Randall, 1989).

CASE STUDY

Sharon's son, Wayne, was 8 at the time of referral. He was in trouble each day at school and had a poor reputation in his home community for aggressive behaviour towards mothers and their small children.

Sharon was convinced that his father's temperament was to blame, even though Wayne had been less than a year old when the relationship failed and the father deserted them both. A psychiatric nurse-therapist made several home visits and observed Sharon alternately shouting at Wayne, then bribing him with sweets, crisps and even slices of meat in order to bring his angry behaviour under her control.

Not surprisingly, Sharon was unable to accept that her management was a significant antecedent to Wayne's challenging behaviour and sought other explanations in terms of food dyes causing attention deficit hyperactivity disorder, the effects of the violent cartoons he watched and the inefficiency of teaching staff. She wanted him on medication because he was 'mentally ill'.

She was gradually reassured that no one thought she was a poor mother because of the difficulties she experienced with Wayne; it was pointed out to her that temperamental differences do exist with children which can make them harder to set limits for and that such children need greater consistency of management as a result.

Parenting style and aggression

Many parents explain that they had wanted to become parents but had been put off by the aggressive behaviour and hostile attitudes of their children. There are several influences associated with such negative feelings about child rearing which cause many parents to respond in ways that are antecedents to their child's later aggressive behaviour. For example, parents respond differently to children who are perceived to be temperamentally 'easy' or 'difficult' (Lytton, 1990), and Kochanska (1993) argues that temperament and parenting style interact strongly to produce undesirable behavioural traits, including aggression. Parenting emotions, beliefs, cognitions and behaviours should be considered alongside background variables including family resources, negative and positive life experiences, the quality of the parents' relationship and the availability of support networks to the parent(s) (e.g. Cox, Owen, Lewis and Henderson, 1989; Rodgers, 1993).

Research also shows that a wide range of stressors on parents are antecedents to the development of aggression within the home. These include economic stress, caused by poverty or the misuse of financial resources (e.g. Weiss, Dodge, Bates and Pettit, 1992; Patterson, 1986; Dooley and Catalano, 1988), marital conflict or conflict between partners (Jouriles, Murphy, Farris, Smith, Richters and Waters, 1991),[1] parental psychopathology including both maternal and paternal depression (Downey and Coyne, 1990; Billings and Moos, 1985),[2] parental substance abuse (Gable and Shindledecker, 1993; Lipsitt, 1990), neurological impairments involving convulsive and memory disorders (Brennan, Mednick and Kandel, 1991), maturational lag in the development of the central nervous system (Monroe, 1974), low-IQ learning difficulties and generally poor academic achievement (Lipsitt, Buka and Lipsitt, 1990).

Authoritative/democratic parenting behaviour is, in contrast, more likely to be associated with the development of mature pro-social behaviour and successful moral reasoning. The children of such parenting style tend to have fairly high self-esteem, be socially responsible, friendly, competent and cooperative, appear generally happy, and be successful academically (Steinberg, Lamborn, Dornbusch and Darling, 1992). This style is in direct contrast with that of parents who provide insufficient or imbalanced responsiveness and control. Those who are authoritarian, permissive or uninvolved are likely to have children who are aggressive and socially incompetent (Lamborn, Mounts, Steinberg and Dornbusch, 1991), particularly when other stresses are present. Cummings (1990) summarises the results succinctly:

> Taken together, then, there is accumulating evidence that preschool children are more likely to show overactive, noncompliant, aggressive and impassive behaviour in the context of uninvolved, rejecting or harsh parenting. Mothers are more likely to engage in these less optional patterns of parenting when they themselves are coping with day-to-day problems in the family and in their lives more generally
>
> (p. 140)

---

1 Jouriles et al. (1991) showed that child aggression is predicted by expressed hostility between the parents, and it is noteworthy that this kind of marital conflict is more predictive of child aggression in boys than in girls (Block, Block and Morrison, 1981).

2 Parental depression does not just reduce positive interactions between parents and child. When the depressed parent is able to take control again it is often found that they did so by becoming extremely authoritative with their children (e.g. Gelfand and Teti, 1990).

CASE STUDY

Jenney looked back on her parenting styles with Robert, her only son, who was placed for four hours each week in a pupil referral unit. He had only a few months of compulsory education left and there was little chance of him rescuing anything worthwhile from them. He was a recidivist bully and there was a prosecution pending after his attacks on an Asian child, half his age.

Jenney reflected that she had seldom had much time for Robert, 'even when he was a toddler'. She commented that she and his father had been too busy with their careers and the latter was often abroad for long periods. Her own work was with a demanding advertising agency and she realised that 'quality time with Robert was in the car coming back from the childminder's'. Whenever teachers had complained about Robert's behaviour, 'all I did was to buy him off with a few little gifts and some words about having to do what he was told. I spent hardly any time trying to understand what was happening or what he was feeling.'

Thus far, parenting styles that are relatively commonplace have been considered. Although they may have their weaknesses such styles are not associated with overt repudiation of a loving relationship between parent and child. What happens when such a situation exists, when children are overtly rejected by their parents and subjected to a style which at best may be neglectful but at worst may be abusive or permissive of abuse by others?

Parental rejection

This is frequently cited by both researchers (e.g. Conger, Conger, Elder, Lorenz, Simons and Whitbeck, 1992) and clinicians (Randall, 1997) as being associated with early childhood aggression. Rejecting parents are more likely to apply power-assertive strategies and punishments (Conger *et al.* 1992). Those parents who are cold, distant and overtly rejecting towards their children, and constantly use physical punishment, are, in common with those whose discipline is inconsistent, more likely to have aggressive children than other parents. Indeed, harsh parental discipline has been found to be a good predictor of child aggression at school (Weiss, Dodge, Bates and Pettit, 1992).

The processes by which parental distance and rejection lead to childhood aggression are complex and the following summary is merely a somewhat crude oversimplification. First, such a parenting style establishes a family environment where feelings of frustration over unmet needs create frustration amongst its members associated with feelings of anger and hostility. These feelings, if left unresolved, are likely to produce hostile and aggressive interchanges between the parents and their children. Secondly, parental rejection and punishment serve as distinctive models of hostility and the inappropriate use of force (Bandura, 1977). Finally, it is also probable that parental rejection constitutes a basis for children to develop an 'internal working model' of themselves as unworthy and of the social world they inhabit as untrustworthy and hostile (Bowlby, 1973). Such negative perspectives and feelings contribute to children's lack of empathy for others in social interactions and to the development of an increasingly refined hostile behavioural repertoire inclusive of bullying. The parents' response to such behaviour represents the beginnings of a circular tragedy because, as they become more rejecting and power-assertive in discipline, so their children respond by even greater aggression (Sroufe, 1988).

Not all parents of aggressive children are cold and punitive, but they apply their power-assertive strategies inconsistently (Parke and Slaby, 1983). Amongst these, some fiercely punish aggression within the home but may encourage it within their children's peer group outside of the home. Some researchers report (e.g. Patterson, 1982) that such parents want their child to achieve dominance within the peer group and will therefore reward such behaviour outside the home inappropriately, even though they suppress it when it occurs within the family.

It is not, however, only parental rejection and punitive behaviour management strategies that result in childhood aggression. At the other extreme, parental permissiveness, indulgence and a general lack of supervision are also antecedents to increases in children's aggressive behaviour. For example, Olweus (1980) found that maternal permissiveness of aggression was the best predictor of childhood aggression. Parental neglect and lack of supervision of children are also known to be related to truancy, precocious sexuality, drinking problems and delinquency in adolescence and adulthood (Lamborn et al. 1991), all of which are correlated with aggression.

Unfortunately, intervention that brings a change in parenting management style does not necessarily lead to a reduction in childhood aggression. Although parenting styles are amongst the best predictors of early childhood aggression, the best predictor for later aggression in adolescence and early adulthood is the persistence of childhood aggression (Eron, Huesmann, Dubow, Romanoff and Yarmell, 1987). This suggests that poor parental behaviour (either rejecting and punitive or uncaring and neglectful) helps to establish a pattern of childhood aggression which becomes the foundation for the development of poorly controlled, aggressive behaviour in later life.

In any event, the older the child gets, the less influence parents have, no matter what their style. During adolescence, the peer group may achieve a strong role in maintaining hostile and generally antisocial behaviour (e.g. Patterson, DeBaryshe and Ramsey, 1989; Cairns, Laung, Buchannan and

Cairns, 1995). It is also during adolescence that some differentiations of antisocial behaviour occur. Thus, for example, bullies tend to have a younger start to their activities than delinquents. This might suggest that bullying is some kind of apprenticeship for delinquency, and that may be true for some individual young people. There does appear, however, to be a differentiation according to experiences of being parented. Baldry and Farrington (2000) suggest that some bullies tend to have aggressive authoritarian parents and disagree with their parents frequently. Delinquents, however, appear to have conflictual and low-supportive parents. It is possible that some bullies who experience distant and inconsistent parenting are those whose pro-social behaviour veers increasingly towards delinquency as they progress through adolescence; the future for them is bleak and they may well be the ones who in adult life fail to develop appropriate attachments with their own children and experience generally dysfunctional relationships.

The effects of being aggressive on the child

Typically the aggressive child develops a sense of being 'bad'. A result of this self-construct is to misread social cues from the interpersonal behaviour of others (Dodge and Frame, 1982). Such children become suspicious and somewhat paranoid, always suspecting the worst. A cycle of reaction is often established away from the parent as well, particularly in school where the aggressive child is likely to become a victim of a negative labelling process (e.g. Hargreaves, 1980). Such a child is very much at risk of social and educational failure and will find few satisfactions within the complex social environment of school. Bullying is often a short-term tactic by which they may gain some satisfaction.

CASE STUDY

Harry was referred for psychological assessment at the age of 14. From the age of 8 years he had been supported in school by specialist teachers from learning and behavioural support services and it was thanks largely to their efforts that he had been retained in mainstream schools.

During his second interview session, Harry revealed that he thought of himself as a 'bad person'. He stated: 'I'm always making life difficult for people – my parents 'specially. They say I'm a bully because I like winding the nerds up; they just get on my nerves and I want to do them over.' When asked how he made life difficult for his parents, he replied, 'They just want an easy life – no problems – I'm just a big problem.'

Harry's parents were older than the norm for a 14-year-old. His father was 62 and his mother was 55; both worked hard and still seemed to be surprised to be parents after many years of a childless marriage. It was noticeable that whenever they spoke of Harry their comments were always preceded by a shake of the head and a puzzled expression, as though they could not believe the type of person that Harry had become.

Bullying his peers was a daily event but he was also disruptive of lessons and regularly failed to observe the rules of team sports during games lessons. He found it hard to defer any form of self-gratification and showed poor attention control whenever he was not being entertained or directed.

Repertory grid work was used to analyse his constructs about relationships. He was found to have a very low opinion of himself as a peer to his fellow students. The constructs he held about his mother were strongly negative, being punctuated by feelings of failed attachment, distancing by her work as a solicitor and being a 'disappointment' to her. Constructs about his father were ambivalent; he sensed positive regard but indicated that communication was poor between them. His support teachers were linked to the strongest positive constructs, and one in particular (who spoke most to him out of lessons) appeared to be given the constructs normally associated with a warm, supportive parent. It was sad to note that Harry expressed fears that he would let this teacher down.

Harry was clearly suspicious of anyone showing him warmth; he tried to bully the therapist working with him by attempting aggressively to get her to make promises about telling his parents how well he was doing. He hoped that they would reward him for this progress by getting him a computer game that he referred to excessively. Harry was surprised and disappointed that she would not collude with him. He would not accept praise for himself but only for the outcome of his actions. For example, he was delighted to be told 'Your story was really well written and I found it very exciting' but reacted angrily on one occasion when he was told 'I think you're a clever boy.' Harry said angrily, 'My parents say I'm bloody thick and the teachers have as well – don't tell me I'm clever, it's just lies.'

The sessions with Harry led to the inevitable conclusion that he was simply acting out as he tested the limits of his distant and generally withdrawn parents. Believing that he was 'bad', he lived up to the self-image he constructed of himself as an unlikeable person. The bullying was one successful way of proving just how bad he could be; it satisfied the criteria he had set to help find stability within his self-constructs.

Chapter 5

Bully characteristics: personality traits

There is a significant amount of evidence that workplace bullies do share personality traits that single them out from non-bullying colleagues and their targets. For example, one research study which made use of grounded theory to explore the subjective impressions of employees on the experience of workplace bullying found that even non-victims perceived them to be loud and to have an overpowering manner which went with a perceived need for power and authority (Mehta, 2000). This resonates with findings from other rather different studies (e.g. Olweus, 1993; Randall, 1997a; Rayner, 1997). Crawford (1992) and Randall (1996), using clinical narrative material, find bullies to have unresolved childhood conflicts, and Weisfeld (1994) describes the high dominance motivation of bullies. In addition, young bullies in the making are unique in that frequently they ignore the submissive behaviour of their victims and carry on inflicting pain (Dodge, Price, Coie and Christopoulus, 1990).

There is also a substantial amount of evidence to the effect that personality factors take second place to organisational variables. Some researchers believe that it is impossible to attribute bullying situations to personality factors. Leymann (1996) believes that it is meaningless to apportion blame to personality once bullying has been detected. Instead, the blame must lie with the organisation for failing to establish proper means of detecting and stopping this behaviour. It is argued, however, that no organisation can be totally effective in preventing all incidents of workplace bullying. It is not always possible to police all types of employment. For example, a small team of men laying cables in an isolated area may be too far from effective supervision. There will often be opportunities for bullying to occur no matter how well-intentioned the managers may be. If the victims are too embarrassed or stressed to report the matter then no procedures will be effective, no matter how superb the background policies may be.

In addition, characteristics of the nature of the employment are known to contribute to workplace bullying. For example, there are some jobs that encourage a bullying style such as sales work and security. Other occupations such as teaching and nursing, are particularly susceptible to bullying situations. Field (1997) argues that professions requiring empathetic staff are more likely to encounter bullying problems because those staff are more likely to be targeted. It is inevitable that any opportunity for the abuse of power means that some people may fall prey to workplace bullies (Olweus, 1993). Despite this series of findings it is still clear that the personality of bullies is an important factor. No one who believes in the fundamental rights of others would subject their work colleagues to the indignity of workplace bullying if they did not have attitudes in support of such behaviour.

Attitudinal factors

Field (1997) has often made reference to the attitudinal behaviour patterns of 'serial' bullies fitting within the diagnostic realms of personality disorder. He characterises the attitude set of such people as marred by selfishness, a need for self-aggrandisement, indifference to the needs of others and compulsiveness about lying, particularly in relation to self-preservation. Field does not profess to have carried out research of an exhaustive and academic nature but his findings were similar to those of the present writer whose clinical narrative studies have been derived from working within employee assistance programmes. It is clear from these studies that recidivist bullies do hold attitudes that allow them to distort events and fabricate criticisms and allegations, demand control over the actions of others in the workplace and believe passionately in their own propaganda. Often clinical interviews reveal attitudes about other people, including the bullies' own family members, which are degrading and completely lacking in empathy. It is not surprising to find, therefore, that many recidivist bullies in the workplace practise similar techniques within their home environment, and attempt to subjugate their children, spouses and partners until they gain satisfaction primarily from the degree of control they exert. Field also suggests that the recidivist bullies' attempts at empathy are superficial and used only for the purposes of improving their image within the workplace. Again clinical narrative studies find some resonance with this when the use of instruments, like the Multimodal Life History Questionnaire (Lazarus and Lazarus, 1991), demonstrates that there is no genuine understanding revealed by empathetic expressions, just a shallow mimicry of other people's concern. Often the same devices reveal insights into the reasons for the recidivist bully's lack of empathy, usually in relation to damaged or dysfunctional parenting, as described in the previous chapter.

Field (1997) links these attitudinal characteristics to psychopathy and from there to a consideration of personality disorders. Whereas there is no substantive research evidence to demonstrate that the majority of workplace bullies do have personality disorders, it is clear that characteristics of these disorders may be present and an understanding of them is vital to the planning of strategies for resolving workplace bullying. In the writer's experience, the formulation of policies and procedures designed to reduce and resolve the personal harassment experienced within a workplace may be successful in alerting many bullies with otherwise normal personality structures to the damage they are causing, such that they stop. Unfortunately, however, those few with serious personality disorders often tend to distort interpretations of the policies and procedures to their own advantage. In a sense, they turn the policy against the employer by refining their bullying behaviour to make it even harder for victims to complain.

Personality disorders

A personality disorder is a stable pattern of inner experience and behaviour that deviate significantly from the expectations of the individual's society. The disorder is pervasive and resistant to change; in most instances the onset is evident in adolescence or early childhood, but causal connections can often be seen far back in the experiences of childhood. Unlike most problems of mental health, the personality disordered individual is relatively stable, although some types are found to remit gradually over the third and fourth decade of life (American Psychiatric Association, 1994). There are several types of personality disorders; two in particular have relevance to workplace bullying; these are Antisocial Personality Disorder and Narcissistic Personality Disorder.

Antisocial personality disorder

This is the personality disorder that most lay people know as psychopathy. In its most brutish forms it has become the subject of lay interest in relation to serial killers and the popular depiction of psychopaths by the media. The onset of this personality disorder is generally to be found in childhood or early adolescence and it continues well into adulthood. Its central features are deceit and manipulation, and therapists working with such people have to avoid being 'charmed' by them into unwitting collusion.

The international classification of mental disorders, DSM-IV (American Psychiatric Association, 1994) provides clear diagnostic guidelines, and forensic examiners of workplace bullies stick closely to these in order to contribute such a diagnosis to the assessment of bully–victim events. For the diagnosis to be given, the individual concerned has to be at least 18 years old and to have had a history of difficult behaviour before the age of 15. This difficult behaviour is often classified as conduct disorder and is characterised by aggressiveness, destructiveness, lying, truancy, poor peer relations, cruelty and rejection of authority and rules. This conduct should also show a definitive repetitive, persistent pattern of behaviour which ignores the basic rights of other people and shows severe violation of age-appropriate societal norms.

This pattern of antisocial behaviour continues into adulthood, and many individuals with antisocial personality disorder repeatedly fail to conform to normal behaviour and find themselves in prison. The majority of these are of low ability and use violence as a means of securing their own ends. The more able may well keep themselves out of prison but nevertheless act in such a way as to disregard the wishes, rights and feelings of others. Deceitfulness is a common trait and they are often highly successful manipulators in order to gain personal profit or power. Their Achilles' heel is often impulsivity, and their presence in the workplace may be illuminated by some unguarded action or comment in front of senior management. They tend to be irritable individuals who are easily aroused to anger and, at the extreme end of the range, they are well represented amongst those who practise domestic violence and the physical abuse of children. At the lower end of the intellectual range of people with antisocial personality disorder are to be found significant impulsivity and irresponsibility. They may become bullies within the workplace but their unpredictability often ensures that they do not remain employed in the same place for very long. Many show significant problems with financial management, failed relationships including parenting dysfunction, high rates of alcoholism and drug addiction, poor work employment records, and incarceration. Typically, they believe that everyone else is to blame and show marked disrespect for victims who appear to be helpless or weak in some way. They minimise the impact of their behaviour on others and many genuinely fail to see how their behaviour could inflict permanent harm.

They are described as individuals with low empathy, callous, cynical and contemptuous with inflated and arrogant self-opinions. Mention is made of their opinionated, self-assured cocky ways and the glib, superficial charm which they use to disguise their true nature and person.

The description of people with anti-social personality disorder also comments that they have problems with monogamous relationships and move rapidly between partners, believing their own excuses as to why the relationships fail. They often act out the difficulties they have witnessed from their own parents and other family members and become increasingly unable to accept normative behaviour and societal rules as relevant to them.

DSM-IV states that the overall prevalence of anti-social personality disorder in normal community samples is approximately 3 per cent for males and 1 per cent for females. The risk to the biological relatives of females with the disorder tends to be higher than that for the biological relatives of males. Males may also develop substance-abuse-related disorders, whereas the females tend towards recurring, multiple and clinically significant somatic complaints (Somatisation disorder).

Not surprisingly, a person with antisocial personality disorder of good ability who can sustain stable employment is quite likely to become a recidivist bully within the workplace environment. Such people can cause extreme damage to others, including psychiatric problems.

CASE STUDY

Gerald was the 31-year-old manager of a regional base of an industrial cleaning company. He was ostensibly charming, witty and courteous. He had a degree in Business Studies and was working towards a post-graduate qualification in management.

Apart from the men operating machinery for dealing with toxic waste, all Gerald's subordinates were women. They were alternately charmed and then repulsed by him and the staff turnover rate was high. His form of bullying was very subtle and completely misunderstood by his remote senior managers.

Gerald's seemingly understanding way was thought to be kindness by women who had personal problems. He noticed signs of stress and encouraged them to talk to him, allowed them to take time off during the working day and generally made them feel valued. He never made any attempt to exploit them sexually and most thought of him as a thoroughly decent person.

Periodically, however, he would target a member of staff and use the information he had about their private life to attack their self-confidence. He gained great satisfaction from pointing out shortcomings in a belittling manner and implied that whatever went wrong for them was simply due to the fact that they were weak, foolish people who asked for trouble and did not have the sense to see it coming. He generally delivered these verbal assaults with a pleasant smile on his face, and some of his victims were unsure on the first occasion of hearing his remarks whether they were being attacked or helped. As he progressed, however, they quickly found that he was exploiting their confidences purely for his own pleasure.

Gerald used his considerable ability to keep his bullying activities away from senior management. Most of his victims simply left the firm and tried to repair their shattered self-esteem elsewhere. Although there were concerns about high staff turnover there was no evidence as to Gerald's part in this. His activities were brought to an end when one of his victims taped his conversation with her. The tape was sent to a senior manager who was horrified by the cold and vitriolic attack on the employee. An investigation led to former employees being questioned and Gerald was revealed to be a very devious workplace bully. He was told to submit to assessment and possible counselling or be dismissed.

Gerald was found to be of high intelligence and socially adept. Use of the Adult Attachment Interview and Multimodal Life History Questionnaire revealed severely dysfunctional parenting including physical abuse, alcohol abuse (both parents) and neglect. His father practised domestic violence and Gerald recalled him beating his mother and saying, 'I'm not going to bruise you where it will show.'

Gerald recalled also how he was sexually abused by a friend of his father around the age of 9 to 11 years. He tried to disclose this to his parents but he was punished and not believed.

On interview, Gerald claimed to have a lot of respect for his father who managed 'to fool everyone into not realising what a swine he really was'. As Gerald moved further into adolescence he deliberately modelled his behaviour on his father who had become a successful businessman; 'If it was good enough for him it will do for me.'

Gerald's bullying began at school where one year-tutor learned that Gerald had become very skilled at lying his way out of trouble. Gerald was proud to have been referred to as 'exceptionally plausible'. The victimisation of younger boys was intense and some parents withdrew their children when they finally became aware of the physical harm being done to their children. Gerald continued his bullying behaviour throughout his adult life. His marriage failed because of it, even though he was quite successful in making out that his wife was an unstable liar. He was convicted of a drink-drive offence, which was the first evidence of severe alcohol abuse. A sudden obsessive interest in weapons led to him being charged with the possession of an unlicensed firearm. He had been impressing people in pubs and clubs by letting his coat fall open to reveal a shoulder holster. When challenged, he claimed that he was in fear of his life after infiltrating a ring of industrial espionage agents.

As part of the assessment Gerald was confronted with his bullying and lying; he denied it all steadfastly and even claimed that the hectoring bullying voice on the tape was not his. He asked the psychologist, 'Do you think I would be stupid enough to let myself be trapped by a stupid woman wearing a wire?' This comment revealed how Gerald lived in some kind of semi-militaristic imaginary world with himself as an unsung hero; his phrases were larded with gung ho Americanisms from films.

Psychometric assessment using the Personality Assessment Inventory revealed particularly high loadings on the scales recording personality disorders. He was eventually diagnosed as having a moderately severe antisocial personality disorder. He underwent a particular type of cognitive-behavioural therapy that is suitable for personality disorder, but even after that was concluded he continued to be unable to understand fully 'what the fuss was all about'.

Narcissistic personality disorder

This personality disorder tends to share a tendency to be tough-minded, glib and superficial, exploitative, and lacking in empathy with the antisocial personality disorder. Most individuals with this personality disorder, however, do not show the characteristics of impulsivity and overt aggressiveness which those with antisocial personality disorder do. Instead, the essential nature of the narcissistic personality disorder is a need for admiration and portrayal of self-importance. These traits, and a distinct lack of empathy, are observable by early adulthood and show themselves in a variety of contexts. In the workplace, these individuals routinely overestimate their abilities and exaggerate their accomplishments. Others see them as being boastful and pretentious and annoy them by not providing the praise and attention they feel their efforts deserve.

It is axiomatic that in order to inflate one's own abilities and excuses, the abilities and successes of others must be perceived as less valuable. Consequently the individual with narcissistic personality disorder is often found to deride the abilities and accomplishments of others whilst being preoccupied with fantasies of their own success, power and value to society. The writer's experience of these people as bullies indicates that they have one common complaint and that is that they have been unfairly passed over for promotion or have had their progress blocked by others who did not appreciate their attributes.

It is not surprising that individuals with this personality disorder fervently believe that they are superior and unique; they expect others to recognise them as such in order to support their otherwise fragile self-esteem. In the workplace, they may tend to persuade others to represent them favourably to senior management, or engineer situations whereby others fail and they succeed.

The writer's clinical work indicates that such individuals are liable to bully their colleagues or subordinates as a means of reducing their own frustration for not rising higher or more quickly within the organisation. Bullying is used also as a means of self-aggrandisement as a consequence of demeaning the efforts of others and/or as a means of proving to themselves that they are more capable, more powerful and more adept in the workplace.

Many are mistaken in that they believe others are very concerned for their welfare and they expect to be listened to frequently and at great length, whilst failing to read the cues that the listeners have their own needs and feelings. Paradoxically, they are quite contemptuous of people who mention their own problems and oblivious to the hurt they cause by giving patronising advice such as 'You'll have to learn to stand on your own two feet.'

Their bullying ways may often come in the form of extremely snobbish, disdainful or patronising attitudes portrayed as rude and deliberately insensitive behaviour.

Although they may not display visible signs of being hurt or otherwise affected, they are extremely vulnerable to the effects of criticism and may dwell on it for lengthy periods. Their reactions are typically disdainful, angry and aggressive; often aimed at the nearest least-powerful individual. Their rise in organisations might be quite swift at the beginning but, as their inability to work comfortably alongside others becomes apparent, so they are increasingly marginalised. Their victims may then get some respite as a result of the long periods of sick leave they are liable to take.

CASE STUDY

Carol at 43 was a Senior Administrative Officer in a local authority department. She constantly chafed at her lack of promotion since she had been given her post eight years previously. She was brought to the attention of the Human Resources department as a consequence of a series of complaints by co-workers who felt picked on, criticised and undermined.

She was accused of being disdainful of her staff and some of the mild-mannered senior officers. Carol lost no opportunity to demean other people's work and patronised juniors by telling them that they may learn eventually but could never expect to reach her skill level. A childless person, she was unwilling to treat anyone sympathetically when they needed a little time for their children, and made sure that she was as difficult as possible.

Whenever promotion prospects arose, Carol endeavoured to damage the reputation of her co-applicants. This merely damaged her own position because her efforts were so blatant. Whenever confronted with her behaviour, Carol became hostile and claimed that she was merely speaking the truth; she knew she was a superior worker and believed that the authority deserved the best. It was clear that Carol relived her own frustrated ambitions by demeaning the skills of others. On assessment she was found to have a high self-esteem but only if she could gain approbation from the clinician. She was alert to the slightest non-verbal clue to possible criticism and began a robust defence which consisted largely of assaults on the skills, appearance and intelligence of her colleagues.

Psychometric profiling revealed a defensive individual with a high level of covert verbal aggression and high egocentricity. A scale recording empathy produced a score approximately 3 standard deviations below the mean. Scales associated with personality disorder were significantly elevated. Not surprisingly Carol would not accept the findings of this assessment.

Failure of empathy

The lack of empathy characterises not only recidivist bullies but also those people with severe personality disorders who may, under conditions favourable to them, become workplace bullies. The capacity for empathy derives from the fact that individuals are able to accept that those around them have equally individualistic thoughts, attitudes, feelings and experiences of pain and hurt. Empathetic individuals are able to respond to the distress of others because they can imagine what it might be like if they experienced it themselves. Bullies hardly demonstrate this humane trait.

The ability to understand the uniqueness of the minds of others is a foundation stone upon which genuine empathy rests, and without that understanding any empathy displayed is nothing more than the sham that Field (1997) has noted amongst the responses of recidivist bullies. Given the consistent clinical findings of low and non-existent empathy amongst recidivist bullies, it seems reasonable to seek an explanation for the behaviour in the ways in which they can conceptualise their social interactions. Randall (1997) reports that many such bullies appear to have no significant awareness of the extent to which their victims feel pain, anxiety, shame and helplessness. The responses of many indicate that they have no understanding that the effects of their bullying persist long after the individual incidents are finished. Randall (1997b) has suggested that these recidivist bullies are lacking in the development known as 'theory of mind', which is of interest to researchers working with children having significant social problems (e.g. Steerneman et al., 1996). 'Theory of mind' has been used by several researchers (e.g. Premack and Woodruff, 1978) to refer to children's developing ability to ascribe thoughts, ideas, feelings, intentions and beliefs to other people and then use this knowledge either to predict or to manipulate the behaviour of these people. For example, lying becomes possible when a child realises that he or she can in some way manipulate the otherwise individual content of another person's mind to believe something that may not be true.

The identification of emotions and that of theory of mind are seen as complementary activities (e.g. Steerneman et al., 1996) because the recognition of emotions in oneself and others is the ability to interpret one's own mental behaviour and that of others in particular contexts. This ability to recognise emotions is seen as fundamental to a developed theory of mind and it is for this reason that researchers such as Baron-Cohen (1989) and others believe that developmental disorders such as autism are characterised by an inability to use theory of mind to develop an understanding of other people's feelings. Without this understanding it is clear that empathy cannot develop. The researchers point out that children can only place themselves in the situation of others if they have developed their understanding of minds being unique but nevertheless able to share common feelings and emotions. In this way the possession of theory of mind enables developing children to give meaning to social behaviour and to modify their behaviour according to their perceptions about how observers are responding to it. This is a form of social insight and reflects an understanding of the social environment which has much to do with the mediation of skilled social behaviour including the portrayal of genuine empathy. It is possible that some bullies who do not fully understand the consequences of their actions, in terms of the long-term pain and distress of the victims, may lack this skill. Some researchers, however, argue that other bullies, often the ringleaders, must have good theory of mind skills to enable them to carry out their manipulations of others (e.g. Sutton, Smith and Swettenham, 1999).

Theory of mind is a developmental skill; that is to say it develops according to the quality and consistency of interactions with others, particularly with one's parents. Just as aggression can be developed as an unwanted trait by unfortunate and damaging parenting experiences, such experiences can also have a profound effect on children's development of theory of mind. It is likely, therefore, that children who fail to establish theory of mind will find it hard to understand the severe and long-term impact of bullying behaviour on others.

Some support for this position is derived from treatment work for people with personality disorders. Young (1989) has developed a cognitive therapy to deal specifically with personality disorder patients and he notes the often extreme rigidity and inflexibility in thought and behaviour which make treatment work difficult. He states (1989) that Early Maladaptive Schemas (EMS) underlie these inflexible patterns and these schemas have to be uncovered and identified. Schemas are regarded as being very stable and persistent having developed during childhood. Their main function is to serve as a template for the processing of later experiences. Young regards them as being unconditional and rigid, often setting extreme standards for the individual to live to. The EMS are thought of in four categories: autonomy, connectiveness (relating to other people), limits standards, and worthiness. These schemas are set down during childhood and are very often the product of dysfunctional parenting. The sheer rigidity of these schemas acts as a block on further social development and this would include the development of empathy and the behaviour associated with it.

Aggressive behaviours associated with these EMS can arise out of the internal triggers provided by them, but they are as likely to be triggered by external events such as the characteristics of particular victims or, indeed, the nature of the organisation in which both bullies and victims work.

The organisation as a trigger

Leymann and Gustafsson (1996) argue that personality determinants of victims may well be consequences of the bullying, and it is certainly the case that the long-term effects of bullying may cause significant changes in the personality structure of victims, often through the processes of traumatic stress. The same comments cannot be made of bullies; it is most unlikely that the actions of bullying in the workplace can create personality variables that are responsible for further bullying, although successful bullying may well 'reinforce' those personality variables that exist already. It is clear, however, that there are organisational factors that are prominent in some settings which would prompt workplace bullying. Leymann (1996) identifies four factors:

1   Deficiencies in workplace design;
2   Deficiencies in leadership behaviour;
3   A socially exposed position of the victim;
4   A low moral standard in the organisation.

Seigne (1998) provided support for Leymann's view. She describes how thirty Irish victims of bullying found their workplace to be highly stressful and competitive, marred by interpersonal conflicts and lacking a friendly and supportive atmosphere. Undergoing organisational changes and management by way of authoritarian leadership style were also important variables. Similarly, as previously described, Einarsen *et al.* (1994) surveyed over 2,000 Norwegian members of six different trade unions and found that both victims and observers at work reported being more dissatisfied than others with their work environment. Responses indicated that lack of constructive leadership, poor opportunities to monitor and control their own work tasks and a high level of role conflict contributed significantly to dissatisfaction. In addition, incompatible demands and expectations around role responsibilities and tasks were thought to cause frustration and stress within work groups, especially when there were difficulties over obligations, privileges, rights and positions.

It was suggested that these difficulties may then act as precursors of conflict, poor inter-employee relationships and scapegoating. Vartia (1996) reported on a Finnish survey and noted that victims and observers of bullying described their work unit as having a poor flow of information, an authoritarian style of settling difference of opinion, poor discussions about goals and tasks and reduced autonomy. Organisational changes brought about precipitately or without a careful consultation process are known to lead to workplace stress, and Sheehan (1998) has demonstrated a link between such changes and workplace bullying.

The author, however, has experienced several situations where these factors have been present within departments as potential organisational triggers but no bullying or other forms of harassment have been reported. It has not been possible to carry out research studies as to why this should be, but personal knowledge of the departments involved suggests that important personality variables defining both bullying and victim potential have not been present.

The author's feelings, without the benefit of empirical research, are that organisational factors act as antecedents to bullying where individuals with pro-bullying personality structures are present. It is important, therefore, to have some model of personality assessment to properly investigate situations where bullying has occurred. The model of workplace bullying given in Chapter 2 deals with this association of personality and organisational variables.

The last chapter examined the significant differences between traits of aggressiveness and those of assertiveness; the distinction enables investigators of bullies to determine, if particular individuals show pronounced traits of aggressiveness, whether or not they are also able to be assertive in an acceptable and pro-social fashion. One of the most critical decisions facing the psychologist or whoever is conducting the examination involves the subject's potential for further aggression. Independently of whether or not legal proceedings are pending, it is necessary to determine whether or not the individual is likely to be a recidivist bully who repeats the behaviour wherever he or she has employment. Unfortunately, this is a very difficult task; psychological measurements have limited success in making predictions about highly specific behaviours within specified circumstances and contexts. This is true also for the prediction of aggressive behaviour generally (e.g. Werner, Rose, Yesavage and Seeman, 1984). The problem is complicated also because of the different ways in which aggression as a construct is represented. Randall (1997a) examined two major categories of human aggressive behaviour and demonstrated that bullying could fall in either or both, as has been described in Chapter 2.

Psychometric evaluation

Although a number of the conceptualisations of the construct are multi-dimensional, it is the case that many of those dimensions are not particularly amenable to measurement. Inevitably, therefore, empirical studies often find that different measurements of aggression do not agree well with each other (e.g. Govia and Velicer, 1985). There have been indicative studies of several multidimensional measures of aggression and one of these, that of Riley and Treiber (1989), examined data from inventories in common usage. These included the rather ancient Buss-Durkee Hostility Inventory through to the relatively modern State-Trait Anger Scale (Spielberger, Jacobs, Russell and Crane, 1983). Factor analysis of the scores from all of these yielded three major factors. The first was a general factor tapping the experience of anger and hostility; the second loaded heavily on to verbal expression of anger; whilst the third was much concerned with physical aggression including fighting and destruction of objects.

It is important that these three factors are examined in relation to bullying behaviour, but, in addition, there should also be investigation of much more covert forms of aggression, which include sub-factors absorbed within the three major factors of the Riley and Treiber (1989) study. Included amongst those would be an additional construct that justifies aggression in order to get ahead or protect one's place in society or an organisation. Running alongside that, but not necessarily related, would be a form of aggression that is not so specifically targeted at particular victims. This occurs when individuals pay no heed to the rights of others and use bullying on an almost daily basis as a standard strategy for gaining ascendancy. Finally, victims who are themselves line managers often suffer from behaviour that is quite passively aggressive but nevertheless damaging. This occurs when individuals appear to be compliant and helpful but actually function covertly to do damage through noncompliancy, rumour-mongering and sowing dissatisfaction.

The Interpersonal Behaviour Survey (IBS) is a valuable psychometric schedule developed to distinguish assertive behaviours from aggressive behaviours and to sample subclasses of these (Mauger and Adkinson, 1980). This questionnaire device carefully delineates between aggressiveness and assertiveness and examines a number of aggressive traits which relate to virtually all forms of bullying that clinical narrative studies reveal.

One scale, the General Aggressiveness Rational scale (GCR), examines the general response class of aggressiveness over a wide variety of item content which includes aggressive behaviours, and feelings and attitudes. Although data are not fully collected yet it appears that recidivist bullies tend to score highly on this scale, whether or not they score highly on the pro-social assertiveness scale. This suggests that many recidivist bullies are prone to the use of aggression across contexts and not just in the workplace.

A second scale, the Hostile Stance scale (HS), evaluated an antagonistic approach towards other people, one where aggression is justified as a means of being successfully competitive and/or to protect oneself against possible threat.

The Expression of Anger scale (AE) is not one that is frequently scored highly on by recidivist bullies. A high score on this scale suggests a person who is prone to losing their temper rapidly and impulsively; many bullies are not impulsive but can successfully hold their temper and bide their time until opportunities are right for bullying behaviour that will not be observed.

The Verbal Aggressiveness scale (VA) is often scored highly on by recidivist bullies who know how to use words to create maximum psychological damage. Items include those relating to criticising, patronising, putting others down and making fun of them.

The Physical Aggressiveness scale (PA) measures the tendency to use physical force in interpersonal situations or to fantasise about the use of such force. Many bullies may have an elevated score on this scale because of their fantasies but never actually put themselves at risk of official action against them by physically assaulting their victims.

The final scale, the Passive Aggressiveness scale (PA), is one that many bully-victims score highly on. It would appear that their consistent behavioural theme in the workplace is one of stubbornness, negativism and complaining, often involving rumour-mongering and derision of the work of others. It is possible that such behaviour draws the individual to the attention of bullies who respond in a hostile manner towards it.

The following case study illustrates the use of this important schedule.

CASE STUDY

Ahmad was referred for assessment at the age of 27. He had a managerial position in a chain of clothes manufacturers and was the cause of a serious complaint of harassment which led his employers to be taken to an industrial tribunal. His bullying had been both verbal and physical and inevitably targeted at women and adolescents.

He was dismissed from the company and was unable to get further employment in his locality. The referral was made by his doctor following a bout of depression. Ahmad denied causing any harassment and blamed his problems on people who were jealous of him. There were no particular indications from his personal-social history and his experiences of parenting and education were satisfactory. His attitudes towards others were, however, very negative and defensive. The clinician believed that this was the result of racial abuse he witnessed towards others during his childhood.

Ahmad took the Interpersonal Behaviour Survey (IBS) and a number of scales were found to be highly elevated. Two of the validity scales were compromised: Denial and Impression Management. The Denial scale concerns a hesitancy to admit to undesirable traits even though these may be fairly common amongst the population. At the highest levels, the scale may reflect serious attempts to distort reality in favour of the respondent. To be in denial is to refuse to accept one's responsibility for a problem by denying all or part of the problem's existence or one's part in it. Unlike any other species, humans can do this because, just as they have the means of representing reality accurately, so they are able to represent reality falsely. As a trait inherent to his language of self-portrayal, Ahmad's attempt at denial made clear that his primary purpose was not to construct a rational model of an alternative to reality where he was not a workplace bully, but to defer conflict; to avoid paying a price for the difficulties, harm and abuse that he was responsible for.

The Impression Management scale is a form of defensiveness whereby the respondent endeavours to present him- or herself as a better person than they are. This is essentially a social facilitation or 'fake good' scale. Ahmad's results indicated strongly that he could not be relied upon to give a true picture of events but sought to create a better but false impression.

Despite Ahmad's obvious attempts to 'fake good' he still showed exceptionally high scores on the General Aggressiveness Rational scale, the Verbal and Physical Aggressiveness scales and the Hostile Stance scale. Assertiveness scales were within the low to low normal ranges. This profile is indicative of a person who has learned to use aggression where assertiveness should be used instead. Unable to accept the wrongness of his social behaviour, Ahmad had never been able to modify his behaviour, and each successful assault on another person simply reinforced his belief that aggressiveness was an appropriate response.

Part 3

Characteristics of victims

Chapter 6

Victim characteristics: personal history and development

The academic study of bullying does little to reveal the deep psychological distress that is experienced by the targets of bullies. Debates about personality characteristics of victims and bullies, the role of organisational factors and the legislative context are vital yet inadvertently they obscure the dreadful anguish that many victims live with year after year. It may be a truism to state that anyone can become a victim of bullying by being in the wrong place at the wrong time, simply by working or living within an environment that fosters harassment and in the vicinity of people who gain positive reinforcement from aggressive activity. Yet, frequently the clinical narratives of those who experience prolonged bullying and suffer the severest of insults to their self-constructs provide an historical dimension to their suffering which extends the span and complexity of antecedents considerably.

These victims are those who experience harassment at different times and in different contexts over a period of years. It may be that their current complaints are firmly rooted in their workplace as it is at the present or of their co-workers as they function now, but investigation of their history often yields a background to bullying that reduces the onus on their employer who would not usually be aware of the extent of their vulnerability. For example, victims of workplace bullying who seek psychotherapy present with a history of severely dysfunctional parenting (Randall, 1997a). In the writer's experience one major group are those who have been subjected to overprotection, or 'smother love' as it is sometimes referred to. The outcome is a social innocence and naivety that is associated with highly dependent behaviour readily evident to potential bullies.

CASE STUDY

Angela was able to write down some of the more significant insights she achieved after cognitive-behavioural work. Amongst these was a final conclusion about her relationship with her father. 'I needed him so much – he was the central figure in my life and I needed no one else but him. It's only now that I realise that he needed me to give his life substance; he lived through me. Every school report, swimming badge and dance class certificate became his achievement through me. When I got my A levels he spoke endlessly to his friends and workmates about them and made them seem much better than they actually were.

'Perhaps if my mother had lived he wouldn't have been so obsessed with me; he used to say that he would be both mother and father but in some ways he was also my gaoler. Children I wanted to be friends with were gently turned away, boyfriends were quickly discouraged by a sort of benign intrusiveness. They gave up easily and I didn't mind.

'I did my degree from home; it wasn't what I'd wanted to study but Dad was so persuasive about it being better to stay at home. It was only when I eventually went out to work that I found I really didn't know how to get on with people. I didn't understand them – they scared me and I thought they were harassing me. I got depressed and Dad thought I should stay at home – I suppose I walked willingly back into the trap.'

Another major victim group is found amongst people from a rejecting parenting style whose parents have been cold, distant and even hostile.

CASE STUDY

Robert provides a description which fits this pattern. 'I was so pleased to leave home but my parents were just as pleased to see me go. I was 16 and had known for years that I was just a nuisance to them. You are supposed to have happy memories of childhood, to feel warm when you reminisce about your parents caring for you. The only warm parenting I ever encountered was the sweet stupidity of "Little House on the Prairie".

'I tried to get alongside my parents but they were too busy carving out careers and fighting with each other to notice me. Misbehaving and getting them called into school certainly got their attention but only for a while before they started bickering about whose fault it was that I turned into a delinquent. The opposite didn't work either, trying hard and being successful at school earned not one word of praise – they were just glad not to have any inconvenient trouble.

'The day came when my father had to sign some papers to let me get into the Army – he never even looked at them, just signed where I pointed and carried on arguing with mother. The Army became my family and I finally found out what affection between people really meant.'

These victims often learn to be submissive in order to avoid serious confrontation and rejection from their parents or siblings, and develop a habit out of this strategy. Unfortunately in later life they find that their submission is a characteristic that potential bullies seek.

These two case studies are illustrative only; they are an oversimplistic representation of processes that are extremely complex and interactive.

> It is seldom the case that any one cause is present, indeed most victims reveal several. Many of them reveal that they have been bullied for years in one way or another and have agonised endlessly as to why they have been singled out for such treatment. In counselling, many gradually disclose other traits about themselves; perhaps as children they cried easily or did not quite fit in; often they were rejected by their peers and not protected by them when they were being bullied; many claim that their parents had not only been overprotective and domineering but were also sexually abusive and most feel that they were in some way denied normal peer relations.
>
> (Randall, 1997a, p. 143)

Vulnerable victims and parental traits

There is less literature on the parenting systems experienced by children who become unassertive victims than there is on those systems experienced by children who become bullies. This is due in part to the fact that shyness, withdrawal and quietness in children are not seen either as 'risk variables' or as indicative of clinical dysfunction. In addition, a pervasive viewpoint was that such facets of personality were biologically determined and not open to significant modification by the socialisation lessons of parents and school (e.g. Plomin and Daniels, 1986). Recently, however, several challenging research studies have emerged in which the phenomenon of social withdrawal, which subsumes the traits of shyness, reticence and quietness, has been revealed to be a variable associated with psychological maladjustment and to some extent predictive of difficulties of internalisation (e.g. Rubin, Chen and Hymel, 1993). This shift of perspective has given rise to further research into the role of parenting and parent attitudes and beliefs about socialisation. The literature takes a wide view of social withdrawal such that many of the characteristics of both child and adult victims of bullying are incorporated. Included are reduced exploration in novel social situations, social deference, timidity, submissiveness, social wariness and anxiety about interactions, and sad affect within peer group contact; also included are negative attitudes about self, including poor self-regard, low self-esteem and acceptance of low status (Hymel, Woody and Bowker, 1993; Randall, 1996).

Although the concept of social withdrawal is too broad to be a precise descriptor of individual victims, it is entirely reasonable to relate it to parenting attitudes and practices that are antecedents to the emergence of victim status. For example, Baumrind (1967) described how children who were generally insecure and unhappy with their peers were more likely to have parents who demonstrated *authoritarian* socialisation behaviours, which created social anxiety and unhappiness, than children who were socially competent. Several studies (e.g. Lempers, Clark-Lempers and Simons, 1989) demonstrated that authoritarian parents employ such styles of child-rearing practices that their offspring develop poor self-esteem, lack spontaneity and show little confidence in social settings. In addition, there are gender effects in that boys, perceived by their teachers to be socially withdrawn, hesitant and spectators rather than participants in the company of their peers, tend to have fathers who are highly directive and less engaging and who show reduced physical playfulness in their interactions (MacDonald and Parke, 1984). This study also revealed that the mothers of these boys tended to be less likely to engage in verbal exchange and interaction. The picture was more confused for girls who show social withdrawal, but in general the parents of socially withdrawn children of both sexes are less spontaneous, less playful and less effectively positive than the parents of socially competent and confident youngsters. When the parents of peer victims of bullying are assessed it is often found that they are under considerable parenting stress. Reliable psychometric instruments such as the Parent Child Relationship Indicator (PCRI) (Gerard, 1994) can be of great assistance. On this test, the profile of these parents sometimes indicates that they get little satisfaction from parenting and that their feelings for their child victim vary on a day-to-day basis. Many subscribe to items which reveal that parenting is not as satisfying as they thought it would be. Parents with the lowest scores on the Satisfaction with Parenting scale dislike many aspects of parenting, seriously question the wisdom of their decision to have a child and experience discomfort with the role of parenting.

This last source of stress is often exacerbated by a perception that the role orientation is different for the other parent. Thus many dissatisfied mothers perceive their husbands to be unsupportive in respect of parenting, leaving them too much with the care of the children.

Another scale that discriminates the stressed parents of child/adolescent victims is the Involvement scale. Low-scoring parents are characterised by emotional distance between themselves and their children. At the lowest end there is little overt concern for the child's welfare and a lack of awareness of the child's preferences, dislikes and activities. On interview some of these parents confirm that they experience high levels of conflict and guilt about the distance between them and their children; nevertheless they feel unable to bridge this gap.

CASE STUDY

Lester was a 33-year-old solicitor who was divorcing his bank-manager wife, Anne, who was having an affair with a partner in the same law firm. They had two children, Sam, 12, and Duncan, 9. Their divorce became a battle ground over property and custody of the children.

Anne had stated that the reason she had an affair was that Lester abused her physically and psychologically. She claimed that he abused alcohol, whilst he counter-claimed that she used cannabis and (possibly) cocaine. Both denied the accusations of the other. Anne's infidelity was, however, uncontested and matters seemed more in favour of Lester for custody although with shared responsibility.

Lester claimed that despite their high salaries they had an expensive lifestyle and were only just able to pay their bills. Anne claimed that Lester was not as successful as he made out and that she had the resources to look after their children properly.

Unfortunately, and largely forgotten by both parents, Duncan was being severely bullied by his peers at school; this was because he was obese and wore thick-lensed glasses. His emotional condition deteriorated significantly but his teachers thought that this was due to his parents' divorce.

As a result of Lester's successful action, Anne was required to take a psychological assessment of her parenting capacity. Her scores on the PCRI were found to be very low in Satisfaction and Involvement, revealing traits of disliking her role as a mother and a wish to be distant from the activities of her children. Her score on the scale for Limit Setting was also significantly high and indicative of strongly power-assertive strategies for behavioural control. In short, she did not want to be a mother or have involvement with her children and was robust in making them obey her so that she could safely carry on with her own pursuits. The fact that Duncan was being bullied was seen by her as character-building and something that he should learn to cope with. She was almost relieved when Lester won his custody application.

CASE STUDY

Julie was the 30-year-old mother of Sally, aged 10, who had severe specific learning difficulties (dyslexia). The father was David, also 30, who was a successful self-employed painter and decorator with two men working for him. The three of them lived comfortably in a semi-detached house in the suburbs.

Sally not only had problems accessing the curriculum but she was being bullied as well. Her teachers seemed powerless to stop the taunting, teasing and physical intimidation (pushing, pulling and tripping up) which occurred on an almost daily basis.

Eventually Sally was removed from school by her parents and family therapy was offered to help her and her parents cope with the stress. As a preliminary to this, both parents were asked to complete the PCRI. Julie's scores were strongly significant on the Autonomy scale and interview confirmed that she did not want Sally to grow up and become more distant from her. The fact that Sally was born after two miscarriages was part of the psychodynamic background to this difficulty.

In addition, however, Julie had a low score on the Communication scale. This indicated a concern that there was only a poor level of communication between mother and daughter. Julie felt that she was unable to help Sally with her problems at school and wanted Sally to come to her to confide in her mother the true depth of distress experienced because of the bullying. Julie believed that she could not communicate effectively on Sally's level and both blamed and overwhelmed her daughter with alternating rejection and over-affection.

By contrast, a second group of parents achieve high scores on Satisfaction and Involvement but low scores on the Autonomy scale. Thus, they are extremely pleased to be parents and show a strong wish to be fully engaged with their children, but fear and resist the normal development of autonomy as their children get older. Those parents who show extremely low scores on this scale indicate some difficulties of over-controlling their children; some admit during interview that they cannot bear the thought of their children growing up and moving away from them emotionally. Some state a wish that their children had remained always in infancy when they were totally dependent and not ready for social play with their peers.

Not surprisingly, these parents may show also a deviant score on the Limit Setting scale which measures the effectiveness and nature of their disciplinary strategies. Their children are left to extrapolate their own rules for acceptable behaviour. Those children liable to become victims are either bully/victims who irritate their peers and attract negative evaluations, or passive conformers who are frightened of many of their peers at school.

Other studies give further support to Baumrind's dimensions of parenting by reporting that children's timidity, social withdrawal and dependency upon adults are strongly associated with overprotection by parents (e.g. Martin, 1975; Parker 1983), a practice which has many similarities in terms of outcome with excessive power-assertion and parental intrusion. In summary, the perception of overprotection is that parents so restrict their children's behaviour that there is less opportunity for social learning outside of the home. The effects of this difficulty are augmented by active reinforcement of dependency. Thus children are encouraged to stay close to such parents who do not reinforce or allow active exploration in novel environments or encourage any form of safe 'risk-taking' behaviours that might lead to the child being psychologically distanced from the parent. Hinde, Tamplin and Barret (1993) have studied preschool children and suggest that the connection between parenting and social withdrawal is not just a matter of the parents' behaviour but also of the children's as well. The data suggested that the children sought their mothers frequently, indicating dependency, and that the mothers responded with reinforcing protectiveness and overly solicitous behaviour. Ladd and Ladd (1994) examined aspects of parenting behaviour and parent–child relationships in association with peer victimisation in young children. Their subjects were 197 American kindergarten children who were videotaped with their primary caregivers in their homes during interactional activities. The behaviour thus recorded was examined as a predictor of peer victimisation. High intrusive demandingness and low responsiveness were associated with increased risk of child victimisation.

Research studies indicate that overprotectiveness is associated with being bullied and the effect is particularly strong for girls who are overprotected by their fathers (Rigby, Slee and Cunningham, 1999). The opposite side of the coin is that low levels of parental care are associated with hostility and bullying (Randall, 1997a). In general terms, low levels of parental care and high levels of overprotectiveness are associated with poor peer relations (Rigby *et al.* 1999). These findings are congruent with earlier research on nineteen dyads of children by Troy and Sroufe (1987) who found that victims of peers often had a history of insecure parent/child attachment patterns. Most victims seemed to have patterns of relating that fitted within Ainsworthy's category of anxious-resistant attachment (Ainsworthy, Blehar, Waters and Wall, 1978). Finnegan, Hodges and Perry (1997) used 184 American children aged 9–12 years and assessed victim status through nomination by peers. The children provided verbal reports about their behaviour and that of their mothers, with particular reference to conflict and control behaviour. Distinct gender differences were revealed. For girls, victimisation was linked to maternal hostility, especially when they were judged by their peers to be lacking in physical strength. It was felt that the maternal hostility might be an antecedent of depression which may have negatively influenced peer group evaluation. Boys, however, seemed to have maternal overprotectiveness linked strongly to victimisation but only in respect of those who were afraid of their mothers and felt compelled to submit to them during conflicts. Finnegan *et al.* noted that although the role of maternal influence was different for each gender, the linking factor is that maternal behaviour does influence children's personal-social development in ways that attract victimisation by peers. Smith and Myron-Wilson (1998) reviewed much of the related literature and concluded that overprotection and family enmeshment were strongly associated with victimisation.

CASE STUDY

Janice was referred to Child and Adolescent Psychiatric Services by her family doctor following a long period of severe bullying during the first year of her secondary school. It quickly became apparent that her difficulties in peer relations extended back to early junior school days.

Her history was one of being a victim of bullying from age 7 on an inconsistent basis. There was a note in the Year 8 records to the effect that her father's overprotection of her made her 'very different from the other girls in the class'. Apparently he even came on to the playground to move her away from games of football because she might be knocked over.

By contrast her mother was found to be distant and unavailable to Janice; family therapists believed that this arose because the father had transferred all his affections to Janice, leaving his wife in an isolated and unwelcomed position.

Existing evidence suggests that the parenting behaviours and styles associated with over-control and overprotection contribute significantly to a broad range of behaviours classified as social withdrawal. Parents using strong power-assertive methods set down many rules and constraints upon their children's social development and create reticent, dependent and timid children who are rapidly targeted for bullying in the playgrounds of their schools. In addition, once away from the source of these constraints, as in the school situation, the children may become unhappy at what must then seem to be a distressing lack of structure, and their expressions of unhappiness may bring them further to the attention of potential bullies. There is also a strong link to sibling bullying as is evident from the research of Duncan (1999) who studied the links between peer and sibling bullying amongst 375 American children. Twenty-five per cent of the children reported being the victims of bullying by their peers and 28 per cent admitted to being bullies. Those children who were bullies and who were also the victims of peer bullying reported the highest frequency of being bullied by their siblings. These are the children who are more likely to have been subjected to punitive, hostile and abusive family treatment than either bullies or victims (Schwartz, Dodge, Pettit and Bates, 1997). Duncan examined also the rate of psychological difficulties amongst the sample and found that those children who had the greatest problems were those who were both bullies and victims. This supports the evidence of clinical studies which indicate that bully–victims are the most likely to suffer long-term psychological disturbance. This is a significant finding because the numbers of such people are quite high; Austin and Joseph (1996), for example, found that they constituted 15 per cent of the sample of 425 children in an examination of the Bullying-Behaviour Scale and the Peer-Victimisation Scale. These rates imply a strong need for intervention and resolution.

It is not difficult to link a social withdrawal outcome of over-control and overprotection to what is known about the characteristics of the childhood victims of bullying. These characteristics have been well researched for over twenty years (e.g. Olweus, 1978). The most common characteristics of childhood bullying victims are those of insecurity, timidity, sensitivity, anxiety and cautiousness. These victims seldom provoke or show aggression and are rarely involved in episodes of teasing. The boys amongst them tend to be physically weak and of small stature (Olweus, 1978). It has been observed by many researchers that such victims do cry readily and attract attention to themselves through this behaviour. Not surprisingly their constructs about themselves are not good and their self-esteem is low with self-beliefs of 'stupid' and 'ugly'. Olweus (1978) labelled them as *passive* and *submissive* because they generally try to placate would-be aggressors rather than assert themselves against them. In later life they describe their childhood at school as lonely with a constant desire for friendship; paradoxically, however, they are not observed to make significant attempts to win friendships. Olweus (1993) demonstrates that their 'submission reaction pattern' contributes significantly to the frequency at which they are bullied.

Olweus (1993) also describes a smaller group of victims whom he calls *provocative* victims. These children are characterised by him as being both anxious and aggressive in the way they react. Their attention control may be poor and they often act in such a way that they annoy other children who become their bullies. It is commonly the case that their high level of activity and disruptive behaviour causes them to be actively disliked by the majority of children in their peer group who sometimes take a pro-bully attitudes along the lines of 'They get what they deserve' (Randall, 1995). This group is very controversial and some researchers (e.g. Smith and Sharp, 1994) have not been able to discover them amongst large sample studies of bullying in school. It is known, however, that the small group of children who are both bullies and victims show the worst outcomes for duration of involvement in bullying and risk of psychiatric disorder (e.g. Duncan, 1999). For example, the work of Kumpulainen, Rasanen and Henttonen (1999) made use of 1,268 8-year-old children who were studied at two time-points using three questionnaires. The children completed the Child Depression Inventory (CDI), their parents completed the Rutter A2 Scale and their teachers completed the Rutter B2 Scale. The results showed that there were significantly fewer female bullies, bully–victims and victims. At a four-year follow-up, the number in all categories had declined and a significant number of children changed status. Thus some bullies became bully–victims and others became victims. Bullying was found to have a significant degree of longevity, however, as almost half of the children found to be bullies at the first study were still involved in bullying four years later. Those who were bully–victims during the first study were likely to still be involved in bullying at the time of the second study. At the time of both studies children involved in both studies showed significantly greater symptoms of psychological dysfunction than other children. Those children from families of low socio-economic status were more likely to be involved in bullying at the time of both studies and to continue to be involved over the four-year period.

The findings concerning backgrounds of victims and bully–victims are encapsulated in the following two case studies.

CASE STUDY: THE PASSIVE/SUBMISSIVE VICTIM

Joel was a 12-year-old boy in a mixed comprehensive school who had been subjected to daily bullying since he was 9 years old. The bullies had moved up with him from primary school and encouraged others to join in their activities.

In appearance Joel was a perfectly unremarkable boy; he was not fat, he did not wear glasses or talk with a lisp. He was white and good at football. Ostensibly he was most unlikely to be bullied but because he cried easily and ran quickly to get adult support he soon brought himself to the attention of potential bullies. Children who liked him stood up for him but because he did not stand up for himself they gradually stopped.

He lived with Mary, a single-parent mother as the father had been killed in a motorcycle accident. She had put all her efforts and devotion into him and hindered his gradual development towards independence as robustly as possible. She acknowledged her overprotectiveness and understood that it was not appropriate. Her stated belief, however, was that he was *her* child and she would bring him up to suit herself.

Mary stopped short of describing him as a possession but it was clear that she viewed him as such. In therapy sessions she was willing to admit that he met many of her needs but only by remaining with her. She squashed any attempts to assert independence and he was frightened of her temper. She compelled him to do her bidding by a mixture of anger and manipulation; she was observed to make him feel guilty for wanting to have peer group activities which would take him away from the home. When this failed she would punish him by becoming angry. Her overprotection was very intense but was backed up by angry shouting, crying and punitive sanctions.

CASE STUDY: THE PROVOCATIVE VICTIM

Kane, aged 10, was referred by his headteacher because of his severe behaviour problems. These included excessively angry responses to provocation by his peers and disruptive behaviour in lessons.

The referral did not mention that Kane was regularly bullied by a group of six boys led by a recidivist bully. When this was uncovered by the psychological assessment, the head and classteacher said simply that he brought it on himself by being provocative. This included making fun of his peers, challenging them to fight and disrupting their playground activities. It was also determined that Kane had severe attention deficit problems. He was unable to concentrate for more than a few minutes on any classroom or leisure activity; any tasks started by him were left unfinished before he moved on to something else and got into trouble.

His parents were dismissive of him and generally issued power-assertive strategies to control his behaviour. His mother often felt guilty because of her attitude towards him; this resulted in a rapid oscillation between angry outbursts and the giving of treats. Both parents were keen on pursuing their own interests and regarded Kane as a nuisance who took up too much of their time. They spent little time with him, told him that he deserved the pain other children inflicted on him and generally neglected his developmental needs. His mother's rapid swings between punishment and promises left him confused and with no clear model of social behaviour. Inevitably conduct disorder and co-morbid attention disorder were diagnosed.

Victim status and the development of interpersonal problem solving

Children behave in their social world as a partial expression of the processes through which they deal with and understand social information (Randall, 1997b). Rubin and Krasnor (1986) suggest a social information processing model which follows a five-part sequence. This is helpful in demonstrating how children who are socially withdrawn develop dysfunctional social skills such that they attract the attention of bullies. Rubin and Krasnor's model suggests that children start the first stage by selecting some **social goal** which involves them in the establishment of some cognitive representation of a desired **end state**. The second stage involves them scanning and interpreting all the cues they consider to be relevant to the social goal, a process referred to as **examining the task environment**. Rubin and Krasnor (1986) show that boys and girls do this differently and arrive at different solutions when faced with the same type of dilemma. In addition, social status, age and familiarity are also strong influences on individual children's goals and strategy selections. The third stage is one of **accessing** and **selecting strategies**, a process that is characterised by the generation of possible plans of action for achieving the social goal and making a judgement as to which are the most appropriate for the given task environment. During the course of the next stage they **implement the chosen strategy**, and in the fifth and final stage they **evaluate the outcome**, a process that requires an assessment of the situation to gauge whether there has been success in achieving the social goal. If the initial strategy has not been successful it may be repeated or a new one may be selected, but under certain circumstances the child may accept failure and abandon all strategies.

When the characteristics of the socially withdrawn child were examined within this model, it was found that preschool and infant children, wanting to acquire some desirable toy from a peer, were more likely than their non-withdrawn peers to show adult dependency behaviours by attempting to engage adults to solve their interpersonal problems (Rubin, Daniels-Beirness and Bream, 1984). In addition, LeMare and Rubin (1987) found that non-withdrawn children were more able to accept the social perspectives of others than those who were socially withdrawn. These findings indicate that the Piagetian-based assumption about the importance of peer group interaction for the development of social cognition is correct in that the socially withdrawn children show clear social cognitive deficits.

Older children, however, were not found to demonstrate the same difficulties as the preschool child. Instead their difficulties were to be found in the production stage of the social information processing model (Rubin, 1985), such that these children attract the attention of potential bullies. The young ones can be easily singled out by their strong tendency to involve adults in getting their own way, a circumstance which even preschool children will object to strongly; and the older ones will behave in a way that draws attention to their vulnerability and immaturity.

It is during middle childhood that regular victim status first becomes evident. It is reasonable to hypothesise that production and enactment difficulties produce a social interaction style characterised by low assertiveness, submission and immaturity. Rubin (1985) has shown that socially withdrawn children are less assertive than their non-withdrawn peers and he also suggests that, when they do assert themselves in an effort to win their own way with their peers, they are more likely to be rejected than socially competent assertive children. Conversely, however, they are more likely to give way to the requirements of their non-withdrawn peers. Over a period of time, therefore, their behaviour shows a steady trait of failed or low assertiveness and ready compliance such that they become recognised as easy-to-bully children. Their problems become more marked with age (Stewart and Rubin,

1995) and more likely to show the 'flattening' of active social behaviour associated with submission (Randall, 1996).

The increasing distancing of these children inevitably leads to poor self-perception and low self-esteem (e.g. Rubin and Mills, 1988). As their childhood progresses, social withdrawal becomes a characteristic trait and they express greater depression and loneliness than their more socially competent peers (Rubin and Mills, 1988). Some research studies (e.g. Hymel, Woody and Bowker, 1993) report that socially withdrawn children aged 10 to 12 years think of themselves as lacking social skills, outside of social support networks and not belonging to their peer group. Many report that being bullied is about the only form of interaction they have with their peer group. Clearly these feelings have a profound impact on the social development of such children and it is inevitable that they influence adult socialisation. For this reason it is possible to trace, for some adult victims, a long history of victim status from their primary education through to the workplace or community.

The transition from child to adult victim status

Many of the regular victims of bullying in childhood are able to withstand their experiences and develop normal social skills for life as adults. Unfortunately many do not, although the exact proportions are not yet clear.

In one study (Coyne, Seigne and Randall, 2000b) of a randomly drawn sample of employees from a large company, approximately 36 per cent of the workplace victims who fitted both Leymann's (1996) definition of mobbing and Randall's (1996) definition of bullying were found also to fall within the most severe category provided by Olweus (1993) as part of the Norwegian national survey. That is, those adult victims reported being bullied once per week or more whilst they were still at school. Of the remaining workplace victims all but approximately 17 per cent reported prior experience of bullying at school of a lesser severity. There appear to be several reasons why some childhood victims are unable to set aside their experiences and become workplace victims. Although severity and frequency of bullying during childhood are obvious factors, which strongly correlate with later submissiveness to dominant and aggressive individuals during adulthood, these variables do not explain those individuals whose experience of bullying was comparatively brief during childhood but who still retain an inability to assert themselves against would-be dominating adults. One hypothesis investigated by this writer is that bullying can cause a variant of childhood post-traumatic stress disorder (PTSD). Unresolved childhood PTSD is known to have significant effects on the development of adult social behaviour and may well act to predispose individuals in adult life to become the victims of adult bullying.

Childhood post-traumatic stress disorder

Clinical studies of children have persistently reported a number of individual post-trauma responses that are consistent with DSM-IV criteria for PTSD. In response to an identified stressor or stressors, children have been reported to show symptoms of re-experiencing (Newman, 1976; Terr, 1979; Eth and Pynoos, 1985), numbing of responsiveness or depressed involvement with external events (Green, 1983) and heightened states of arousal (Burke *et al.*, 1982).

Increased vulnerability to PTSD is found in traumatised children, particularly those under 11 years, and adolescents (Davidson and Smith, 1990; Pynoos and Eth, 1985). Both groups experience psychosomatic complaints, including headaches, visual and hearing problems (Pynoos and Eth, 1985), school avoidance, concentration problems, weak academic performance, sleep disturbance such as insomnia, frequent waking, night terrors, bed wetting and somnambulism, withdrawal, suicidal ideation, appetite disturbances (Davidson and Baum, 1990), memory impairment, irritability, hypervigilance, exaggerated startle responses, outbursts of aggression, avoidance of trauma-related stimuli (Amaya-Jackson and March, 1995; Terr, 1995), and suspiciousness (Terr, 1995).

Although early reports were inconsistent in the selection of individual symptoms reported, there has been a significant demonstration over the past decade that there is the same relationship between the proximity or degree of exposure to a life-threatening event or other trauma and subsequent levels of symptoms or degrees of impairment for children as there is for adults (Pynoos, Frederick, Nader and Arroyo, 1987). The DSM diagnostic criteria for PTSD are based around the following major cluster of symptoms:

1   Exposure to an event that would be considered traumatic for most people;
2   Intrusive re-experiencing of this trauma;
3   Numbing of responsiveness to or reduced involvement with the external world which may include an inability to recall an important aspect of the trauma;
4   Persistent evidence of hyper-arousal.

Since many of these symptoms overlap with other diagnostic categories, most particularly in respect of depressive disorders, anxiety disorders and various adjustment disorders (Jones and Barlow, 1990), the application of these criteria to children has been controversial, and doubts have been expressed that children manifest symptoms of PTSD in the same way that adults do (e.g. McNally, 1991). One of the ways in which children with PTSD may differ from adults with PTSD is in the nature of traumatic re-experiencing (Nader and Fairbanks, 1994). There are reports that children arc less likely to re-experience the kind of dissociative flashbacks that adults commonly report. For example, Lipovsky (1991) reports that children more typically have re-experiencing symptoms in the form of nightmares that relate to the traumatic events.

Further differences from the adult version of PTSD have also been raised in terms of the possibility that children suffer not one but two types of post-traumatic stress. On the basis of extensive clinical observation, Terr (1989) has proposed Type I and Type II childhood PTSD. The first type results from a single-impact traumatic event whereas Type II is the product of a series of traumatic events or prolonged exposure to a particular stressor or stressors. Terr claims that Type I PTSD does result in children having the classic re-experiencing symptom, whereas Type II PTSD is more commonly typified by dissociation, numbing and denial and may be associated with the subsequent development of multiple or dissociative personality disorder. If this topology is an accurate reflection of PTSD variation amongst children then it is of particular relevance to clinicians who work with them therapeutically.

It is reasonable to assume that the experience of bullying may provoke both Type I and Type II PTSD. A very severe encounter with a bully may be a sufficient single-impact trauma to provoke a Type I response and, alter-natively, Type II responses may be provoked by regular and severe exposure to bullying. In both cases the children involved would require therapeutic intervention designed to alleviate the effects of PTSD in order to reduce the associated long-term difficulties; it is unlikely that simply treating them as the victims of bullying would have the same beneficial effect.

Aggression and childhood PTSD

Some of the best studies linking the experience of aggression to PTSD in childhood come from observations of children exposed to risk in war zones. Recent studies (e.g. Elbedour, Ten Besel and Maniyarna, 1993) concern chil-dren of the Middle East conflict, and research is currently ongoing on the effects of the Bosnian war on young children. Elbedour *et al.* report that the children of the Middle East conflict have developed a wide range of symptoms, including fear, depression, anxiety, anger, phobia, restlessness and other difficulties. They estimate that at least 21 per cent of the children in Gaza face the risk of developing severe mental health problems within the clinical range, whereas, in the United States, only 5 per cent of children sampled by the same instruments fell within that range. These children were exposed to both single-impact and sustained aggressive trauma. It is reason-able to expect, therefore, that they would show evidence of both Type I and Type II PTSD according to Terr's (1989) description.

Some single-impact traumatic incidents have been studied. A particularly good example is that given by Pynoos *et al.* (1987) in respect of 159 children who were subjected to a short but intense trauma when a sniper opened fire on their school yard. The use of a Child PTSD Reaction Index revealed, on analysis of variance, significant differences by exposure but not by sex, ethnicity or age. Additional analyses of individual item responses, overall severity of the PTSD reaction, symptom groupings and previous life events showed strong evidence that acute PTSD symptoms can occur in school-age children, with a significant correlation between the proximity of the violence witnessed and both the type and number of PTSD symptoms.

Victims of school bullying show behaviours that mimic those of adult sufferers of PTSD (Ambert, 1994; Branwhite, 1994; Randall, 1997; Rigby, 1997; Sharp and Thompson, 1992; Smith and Sharp, 1994). These behaviours indicate that bullied students may have a relatively increased vulnerability to post-traumatic stress disorder. Hawker and Boulton (2000) reviewed cross-sectional studies of the association of peer victimisation with psychosocial disturbance. They reported that victimisation was more closely associated with depression than with anxiety and concluded that there needs to be further and more involved research into the cause and treatment of victims' distress. It is clear, therefore, that persistent victimisation in childhood and adolescence will result in severe psychological harm at the level of psychopathology and for which treatment is necessary.

These and similar studies reveal a consistent PTSD response to exposure to violence, and lend credibility to the belief that bullying, as a personally experienced variety of aggression, could also lead to the manifestation of post-traumatic symptoms. In one study the writer surveyed 290 primary school children, aged 9–11 years. Of these 12 per cent claimed to be bullied once per week or more frequently. The responses of these children to a modification of the Post-Traumatic Stress Inventory (Pynoos et al., 1987) revealed that over 75 per cent experienced significant post-traumatic stress effects. A further 5 per cent of the total sample also scored within the pathological range on the test despite a lower incidence of being bullied. These data not only confirm that bullying can lead to severe post-traumatic effects but also support the belief that bullying can be both a Type I and a Type II stressor.

Given what is known about the relationship of unsuccessfully treated PTSD in childhood and later adult problems of mental health and adjustment, it is therefore reasonable to suppose that an inadequate or inappropriate response to the victims of bullying may result in later problems during adulthood for those victims. This is congruent also with work on the victims of childhood abuse and their later vulnerability (e.g. Frederick, 1985).

Chapter 7

Victim characteristics: personality factors

The last chapter outlined some of the developmental histories and dysfunctions of socialisation experienced by many victims of childhood and adult bullying. It is inevitable that such dysfunctional experiences would be reflected in adult personality characteristics, some of which may predispose individuals to being the targets of bullying in adulthood. Evidence will be presented that the personality structures thus formed are associated with stable patterns of interpersonal behaviour which may become the antecedents of bullying in the workplace. In this chapter, the personality structures found amongst some victims are considered and also those structures that are associated with people who are bully–victims. This refers to those people who are victims of workplace bullying but who are also the source of bullying experiences to others.

The victim and the bully–victim

The demarcation drawn by Olweus (1978) between submissive and provocative child victims is relevant here also. As described previously, the most common characteristics are those of cautiousness, sensitivity, anxiety and insecurity. These victims do not provoke, tease or show aggression and may have special needs. When confronted by bullies they often cry or show other obvious signs of their distress. Their self-esteem is low and they feel as negatively about themselves as others do and frequently describe themselves as stupid or ugly. Olweus has labelled them *passive* or *submissive* because they seek to placate rather than be aggressive in response.

In contrast, there is a smaller group of victims whom Olweus labels *provocative* victims. They have both anxious and aggressive reaction patterns. They may have poor attention control and act in such a way that they annoy other pupils who become their bullies. It is commonly the case that their overactivity and disruptive behaviour cause them to be disliked by most children in their class.

This last factor is highly significant because there is often a loss to the provocative victims of peer group support. In fact, although the attitude of children is generally pro-victim, this is not the case in respect of provocative victims. Indeed, there is considerable evidence that young people want to distance themselves from these victims and believe that they get what they deserve. Such young people may conceptualise some aggressive behaviour, which adult observers refer to as bullying, as a punishment meted out by the more powerful on the undesirable (Randall, 1995). The lack of peer support to the victim tends to prolong the period over which bullying occurs. It is also the case, in the author's experience, that teachers will turn a blind eye to the bullying punishment of such pupils because they hope that the peer pressures will act to modify the offending victim's behaviour.

Although some researchers have failed to identify the provocative subtype victims, others have been able to identify students in school situations who function both as bullies and victims (e.g. Austin and Joseph, 1996). As has been stated previously, those children who are both bullies and victims tend to show the highest levels of psychological difficulty (e.g. Duncan, 1999) and, in respect of adolescent males, come from families where there are reported significantly lower levels of affect and communication than for other students (Rigby, 1994).

Clinical narratives resonate well with a proposal concerning the extension of the concepts of submissive and provocative victims into workplace settings. The clinical narratives accumulated by the author do support Leymann's (1992) view that the bullying process starts from a conflict, and give credence to Thylefors (1987, cited by Einarsen, 2000) who describes bullying as a complicated interactive process in which the organisation, the group, and the victim have specific roles. In addition, Leymann (1992) also identifies that bullying at work is related to the type of work undertaken. Thus people working in administration and public services were subjected to mobbing with a higher frequency than those engaged in research, teaching or production work. It is inevitable, however, that personality factors are implicated as potential sources or contributory influences in respect of conflict. For example, Brodsky (1976) described victims as tending to be conscientious, literal-minded, somewhat unsophisticated, and presenting sometimes as underachievers with an unrealistic opinion of themselves. She states that some victims of harassment are rigid, sometimes paranoid, and others are compulsive. Evidently organisational and occupational factors appear to be antecedents for the development of conflict and the presenting personalities of the victims provide information for 'targeting' by bullies.

Personality traits and targeting

Much of the research work relating to this has been carried out in school settings. Thus, for example, victims of school-based bullying were found to be lower in extroversion and higher in neuroticism than control pupils (Byrne, 1994; Mynard and Joseph, 1997; Slee and Rigby, 1993). In addition, submissiveness and sensitivity are associated with a higher risk of being bullied at school (Olweus, 1993; Schwartz, Dodge and Coie, 1993).

O'Moore, Kirkham and Smith (1997) presented results of an Irish nationwide survey of bullying behaviour in primary and post-primary schools carried out during 1993–4. A total of 20,442 pupils from 531 schools in the Republic of Ireland took part and data were presented on the incidence of bullying and being bullied, year differences, gender differences, types of bullying, where bullying occurred, pupil attitudes to bullying and teacher/parent awareness. Amongst the wealth of results 14.1 per cent of the sample were identified as bully–victims as compared to the 12.3 per cent who were bullies only and 17.1 per cent who were victims only. Austin and Joseph (1996) surveyed 425 children (204 boys and 221 girls), ranging in age from 8 to 11 years, in order to develop two self-report scales (the Bullying-Behaviour Scale and the Peer-Victimisation Scale) to assess bully/victim problems at school. These scales were designed so that they could be located within the Self-Perception Profile for Children (SPPC). Their data indicate internal reliability of both scales as being satisfactory. Showing some small variation from the O'Moore et al. study (1997), Austin and Joseph reported that 22 per cent of their sample were classified as victims only, 15 per cent as bully–victims, and 9 per cent as bullies only. Pure victims were reported as being less forthcoming, more withdrawn, and more neurotic than both bullies and controls. Bully–victims tended to have lower scores on behavioural conduct and global self-esteem measures.

Mynard and Joseph (1997) reported on a study of 179 children ranging in age from 8 to 13 years who completed the Bullying-Behaviour Scale and the Peer-Victimisation Scale from the Austin and Joseph study (1996), the Self-Perception Profile for Children (SPPC), and the Junior Eysenck Personality Questionnaire (JEPQ). Their results provided figures for bully victim classifications similar to those of Austin and Joseph. Eleven per cent were classified as bullies, 20 per cent as victims and 18 per cent as bully–victims. There were marked variations on the JEPQ results in that bullies scored lower on the lie scale, victims scored lower on the extroversion scale and bully–victims scored higher on the neuroticism and psychoticism scales than children who were not classified as involved in bullying. These results show a very complex personality structure for bully–victims in childhood which certainly delineates them significantly from bullies only and victims only. It should be noted that these characteristics are persistent and are likely to remain so until adulthood.

Randall (1997b) reviewed the pattern of scores on the Devereux Scales of Mental Disorders (DSMD) completed by the parents of child victims, bully–victims and bullies aged between 8 and 12 years. These scales are used to identify psychopathological and behavioural problems in children by providing a measure of overt problem behaviours exhibited by individuals. The scales provide an overall score and give separate scores for factorial-derived subscales which reveal the major categories of psychopathological symptoms. There are three broad composite factors: Externalising, Internalising and Critical Pathology. These are derived from separate scores on subscales of Conduct, Attention, Anxiety, Depression, Autism and Acute Problems.

Analysis of the results is strongly indicative of differentiating pervasive personality traits even at this age. The regular bullies scored highly on the externalising behaviours, showing traits of aggressiveness, regular annoyance to others, class and family disruption, restlessness and, for some, inattentiveness. Their score on the conduct scale was significantly elevated, revealing traits of disruptive and hostile behaviour in addition to their aggression.

The bully–victims tended to be less externalising but their scores on the conduct scale were equally as elevated as those for bullies and showed a significant tendency to violate the basic rights of other people (usually their peers), impulsivity and disregard of the norms of age-appropriate social behaviour. There are strong associations here with the findings of Mynard and Joseph (1997) of high scores for bully–victims on the Psychoticism scale of the Junior Eysenck Personality Questionnaire (JEPQ). In addition, the bully–victims had elevated scores on the internalising composite, revealing poor self-esteem, anxiety and lowered mood. It would appear, therefore, that many bully–victims tend towards mixed emotional-conduct disorders.

By contrast with the bullies, the regular victims showed excessive worrying, social withdrawal, anxiety and over-control. They experienced high levels of tension, low self-esteem and psychosomatic complaints. In short, they are rather like their adult contemporaries as described by Zapf (1999). It was noticeable, from the pattern of items scored by their parents, that these children had already begun to withdraw from social contexts, and showed reduced interest in age-appropriate activities. Avoidance behaviours (e.g. towards school) were common. Randall (1997a) reported that parents identified consistent traits amongst their child victims including:

- appearing discouraged or depressed
- not showing joy or gladness at a happy occasion
- remaining alone or isolated
- appearing uncomfortable or anxious with others
- refusal to go to school
- withdrawal from or avoidance of social contacts
- becoming easily upset
- telling lies
- having difficulty sleeping
- showing a strong fear of rejection
- showing an exaggerated fear of getting hurt
- appearing sleepy or tired during the day
- becoming distressed when separated from parent/guardian
- demanding physical contact from others

- getting startled or acting jumpy
- clinging to adults

This author (Randall, 1997a) made the point that these behavioural items are indicative of the developing victim personality and are associated with other specific behaviours that are the consequences of avoidance strategies. These include:

- going to and from school by long routes
- appearing nervous and jumpy around other children
- stealing from home to 'buy off' bullies
- having relationship problems in the peer group
- mysterious aches and pains, vomiting

The plight of one young child typifies the victim profile identified by the DSMD results:

CASE STUDY

Steven, at the age of 10 years, was referred to the Education Welfare Officer because of his poor attendance at school and minor delinquency when he should have been attending. He said he was not being bullied but his friends and a cousin had witnessed it.

Often he came home late from school and made excuses that he had been helping the caretaker. He often returned in filthy clothes and his watch and pens were broken. In common with many young victims he began stealing from his parents in order to give money to the bullies and he had often had to steal from his siblings as well.

He was bed wetting frequently, scarcely ate, complained of feeling sick and developed sleep disorder. Steven began to experience random psychosomatic symptoms and became both overactive and hypervigilant. He showed increasingly reluctance to separate from his parents and full school refusal followed inevitably.

On the basis of clinical narrative studies, Randall (1997a) suggests that the differentiating traits are likely to emerge in adulthood and so create adult personality structures associated with bullying or being bullied. O'Moore, Seigne, McGuire and Smith (1998) gave a sample of thirty self-selecting Irish workplace victims the 16PF. The mean scores were lower amongst the victims than the 16 PF norm group for Emotional Stability and Dominance, as well as higher in Anxiety, Apprehension and Sensitivity. The victims tended to be more neurotic, anxious and with low levels of self-esteem. Einarsen, Raknes and Matthiesen (1994) discovered that victims in a Norwegian survey believed that they lacked coping and conflict management skills and that their shyness contributed to being bullied.

Zapf (1999), in a paper advocating the multi-causal nature of mobbing, argues against one-sided explanations of the phenomenon. The detailed research that this paper reports provides invaluable insights into the causes of bullying at work and extends our knowledge extensively over organisational and occupational issues. In addition, however, the findings suggested that some of the reasons for the mobbing were perceived to lie in the victims themselves. Zapf is careful to point out that one cannot blame victims for being victimised any more than, under certain organisational circumstances, one can blame people for becoming bullies. Although victims appeared to have an almost naive belief in their own efficiency at work, well above that which one would expect, they did identify in themselves an inability to recognise conflicts as quickly as their peers. Several items distinguishing victims from others referred to a lack of social skills and weak unassertive behaviour. Not surprisingly the group shown to be high in unassertiveness and avoidance reported significantly higher levels of anxiety and depression compared with the other groups. The victim group showed a significantly higher level of negative affect than a control group who were significantly lower in respect of psychosomatic complaints than all the other groups.

Anxiety, depression and negative affect are strongly related to neuroticism, whereas psychosomatic complaints are a general stress indicator which may be independent of such a long-term personality characteristic. Zapf believes, therefore, that there is a group of individuals who have pre-existing symptoms of anxiety and depression and negative affect with lower social skills and efficiency in social behaviour such that they are even more likely to become victims of mobbing. They share a trait of conflict avoidance and, where this avoidance is impossible, tend to be submissive. Another group of mobbing victims, however, showed no significant differences from the control group except in respect of psychosomatic complaints. This suggests that they were free of pre-existing conditions but experienced mobbing anyway and so became severely stressed. Not surprisingly, those victims who have the pre-existing conditions are the ones most likely to need psychiatric or psychological help. Zapf suggests that those victims who did not have pre-existing conditions and did not develop anxiety and/or depression as a consequence of the mobbing may seek to relieve their stress (recorded as elevated psychosomatic complaints) by seeking employment elsewhere. As a result they are less likely to come into contact with psychologists or psychiatrists and so perpetuate something of a myth that victims are people with vulnerable personalities. Nevertheless, there is a clear link between personality variables and victim status which has to be taken into account.

Vartia (1996) stated that there is need for further investigation into the role of personality in workplace bullying, particularly at the stage when victims are targeted. Vartia suggests that they may be selected as a consequence of their personality because potential bullies seek weaknesses such as conflict avoidance, submissiveness and a lack of social skills. Inability to cope (Einarsen, 1999) may be a further reason for targeting by potential bullies – for example, a child who cries readily at school. In addition, some victims may provoke aggressive behaviour from bullies (Einarsen *et al.*, 1994). Clinical narratives strongly support the views of Zapf and Vartia. The following case studies are illustrative of a victim who had pre-existing vulnerabilities and another who had no such difficulties but who became stressed as a consequence of institutional bullying.

CASE STUDY

Jill, aged 27, took a job as a civilian librarian in a major drug company. She was one of a group of people who catalogued drug trials for the company and cross-referenced them to research studies from around the world. It was also part of the job to access research and clinical studies on a big range of medical disorders that the company was interested in.

She had had moderate problems of anxiety and post-natal depression in the past; she had also experienced significant verbal bullying whilst in secondary school. From that time on she was unaware that she was on a constant lookout for people making derogatory remarks about her. Jill believed that questions about what she was doing were thinly disguised criticisms and that disagreements about procedures were attacks on her competence.

Not surprisingly, her responses to these perceptions drew her to the attention of her colleagues. They grew exasperated with her and two in particular were openly hostile. Jill took their hostility as confirmation of her original perceptions of harassment and began to be covertly critical of the two co-workers behind their backs. She complained frequently about them and eventually this created antecedents for robust negative evaluations by them. This led to genuine harassment as the unresolved conflict dragged on; no one supported Jill as most believed that she had simply brought the problem on herself.

CASE STUDY

Jim was a 40-year-old training officer who had worked for many years in the training division of an electronics company. He was made redundant when it was taken over and promptly found himself a post as training officer in an NHS Trust. People said that the speed with which he made the transition at work was typical of him – intelligent, stable, good-humoured and 'laid back'.

He had only been in the post for a matter of weeks before he found that all his work was being given to a co-worker of equal status. She had been told by their manager to 'keep a close eye on Jim'. He accepted this for a few weeks until he noticed that his work was actually superior to that of the co-worker. He spoke to his manager about this and she was affronted. From that time, Jim found himself to be increasingly harassed by her. He was given clerical jobs to do and impossible dead-lines. His computer was removed and he was expected to share one with trainees in the department. Vital information was kept from him and he failed to deliver an important training pamphlet on time because he had been given the wrong deadline. He decided to go 'off sick' until such time as he found a different job. He felt this was a far easier option than trying to stay in a hostile sub-culture where the work standards were well below his own.

What then is the significance of personality structures that may delineate victims from non-victims? Leymann (1996) believes that personality charac-teristics may develop more as a result of being bullied rather than be an antecedent to bullying. On the other hand, Vartia (1996) has argued that personality factors could be of importance at this stage when the victim is targeted by individual bullies. Clearly, if potential victims do bring with them a particularly vulnerable personality type to the workplace, then there are important ramifications to how they are dealt with by managers. It may be that the victim personality profile, if it exists, is indeed created by the effects of bullying, but this could have a lot to do with prior experiences of bullying during childhood, perhaps at school, in the community or by siblings at home. Clearly, childhood is the time when personality structure is fluid and environmental influences impact on it greatly. The traumatic effect of being bullied regularly would be a powerful influence on personality development. At one level, therefore, Leymann and Vartia could both be right. Bullying may well create a predisposition to victim status in childhood which is then brought to the workplace. Two significant questions exist, therefore: first, is there such a thing as a victim personality profile which may predispose a person to being bullied in the workplace; and secondly, is there evidence that people possessing this profile have had significant prior experiences of early bullying? The second question has already been examined in the last chapter where strong evidence was found of significant prior experiences of being bullied at school. The study described below (Coyne, Seigne and Randall, 2000a) represents a unique attempt to deal with the first question.

Victim profile

Samples

Data for this study came from 120 employees, made up of 60 victims and 60 non-victims. Both samples, from two large organisations, were of people from different areas, having a broad range of backgrounds, representing different professions and occupations in the public and private sectors of the Irish workforce. The first sample came from a large public organisation with a workforce of approximately 1,500 employees. A broad range of employment types included personnel, engineering and clerical. The sample comprised 30 males and 30 females from 10 different departments. The age distribution was: 41–50 (40 per cent); 31.7 per cent were between 31 and 40; 15 per cent between 25 and 30; 11.7 per cent between 18 and 24; and only 1 was in the 51+ group. Respondents were matched in terms of gender, age and occupation (see below).

The 60 respondents from the second sample came from a private multinational organisation with a workforce of about 1,300 at the selected site. Once again, a broad range of employment included sales, marketing, production and management. Although many of the victims/non-victims were matched in terms of the criteria outlined previously, some differences did occur in gender, ages and employment grades. There were 34 males and 26 females in the sample and ranges were: 31–40 (30 per cent); 28.3 per cent were in the 41–50 range; 21.7 per cent in the 25–30 range; 15 per cent in the 51+ range; and only 3 people in the 18–24 range.

Design/procedure

Several meetings with management and unions took place in order to gain permission to interview employees. Management was informed throughout the survey. Initial contact with most of the respondents was made in the canteen area during meal breaks and the aims of the study were described. An explanation was given that the study needed data from the respondents (whether or not they had been bullied) which would be obtained by an interview about their working and social environments. At this point a personality questionnaire was distributed. Participants were asked to complete the questionnaire by themselves in their own time. Contact numbers were taken, and a suitable time for interviews was arranged for their respective departments.

The interview schedule consisted of approximately 30 questions (open and closed) which were subdivided into 6 sections: personal; work details; bullying behaviour and its effects; present home; community; childhood environment. At this stage the victim and non-victim groups emerged according to the following definition of bullying:

> When a person is bullied in the workplace, he/she is repeatedly exposed to aggressive acts, which can either be physical, psychological and/or verbal. It is where cruelty, viciousness, the need to humiliate and the need to make somebody feel small dominate a working relationship.

The interviewer asked each participant if they were exposed to this behaviour and if so for how long and to what extent. Those who had been bullied in accordance with Leymann's (1992) time-scale of aggressive acts that occur on at least (statistically) a weekly basis, and over a period of more than six months, were classified as victims. They were then asked if any of their colleagues were bullied. Positive responses allowed the interviewer to seek these persons to see if they would cooperate. In this way the victim group was established.

Near-match colleagues who were not bullied were identified in terms of gender, age and job status. A near match was also applied for the non-victims' marital status, community and social environments; in this way the control group was established. In some cases, it was the non-bullied individuals who were interviewed first and the interviewer (using the same format) then searched for bullied colleagues.

All respondents were given an assurance of confidentiality for all stages of this study. The interviews were conducted in a semi-structured manner with the help of a schedule. This format allowed expansion and exploration of some of the issues that arose during the interview in order to obtain a richer picture of the respondent's work and personal-social life history.

Materials

The ICES Personality Inventory (Bartram, 1994) was used as a suitable work-related personality test. The ICES examines four major scales (Independence, Conscientious, Extroversion, Stability) which closely map on to the 'Big Five' factors; within each major scale are two minor scales. The major scales of ICES are factorially distinct whilst the minor scales are conceptually distinct; they are designed to provide richer descriptions of personality differences. A description of the scales is given in the appendix to this chapter.

Independence (I) refers to the extent to which an individual is single-minded and determined to win, at one end, as against likeable, diplomatic and submissive at the other. The Competitive minor scale (I1) focuses on the single-minded/cooperative dimension and the Assertive scale (I2) on the outspoken/conflict avoidance one. Conscientious (C) assesses traits such as rule-abiding, moralistic, traditional, organised and dependable. The two minor scales are Conventional (C1), which examines the conventional/flexible dimension, and Organised (C2), which examines the orderly/creative one.

Individuals scoring high on the Extroversion (E) trait tend to be sociable, outgoing and often seeking excitement, whereas low scorers are content to be alone in familiar surroundings. The minor scale of Group-oriented (E1) reflects the extent to which an individual needs approval and support from other people, and the Outgoing (E2) minor scale (E2) reflects the extent to which an individual is talkative, impulsive and the centre of attention. Stability (S) examines whether an individual tends to be relaxed and stable, at one extreme, as against anxious, easily upset and irritable at the other. The minor scale of Poised (S1) examines the extent to which an individual can easily shrug off criticism and cope with adversity, and the Relaxed (S2) minor scale reflects the extent to which an individual tends to be untroubled and calm. In addition, ICES also has a Social Desirability scale which indicates if an individual has been frank in their responses. A high sten score of 9/10 is usually considered an indicator of a possible distorted profile.

There is evidence of good content and construct validity. ICES has been shown to correlate strongly with the 16PF (Bartram, 1993) and the Hogan Personality Inventory (Bartram, 1998). Internal consistency reliability co-efficients range between 0.6 and 0.85, and test-retest coefficients over a one-week interval range from 0.60 to 0.86.

Results: sample 1

Means and standard deviations of the sten scores on the ICES scales were obtained for the development of both samples. An independent t-test was used to determine if differences were significant at or beyond the 5 per cent level.

Initially, examination of the means and standard deviations for the ICES sten scores in the non-victims in both samples revealed them to be representative of the norm group of working adults on the majority of scales. Given that the non-victims were not significantly different from the norm group they can be considered an appropriate control group.

For sample 1, significant differences between victims and non-victims on all ICES major scales were found. The largest difference was on Stability, where the victim group's mean sten score was at the extreme end, indicating high levels of instability, anxiety and neuroticism. Those low in Stability tend to be 'anxious, suspicious, sensitive and emotional and may have problems coping with difficult situations' (Bartram 1994, 1998, p. 144). Analysis of the difference between the groups on the minor scales of Stability (S1-Poised and S2-Relaxed) shows the same pattern as for the major scale.

A highly significant difference emerged for Independence, with victims revealed as less assertive, competitive and outspoken than non-victims. When examining the difference on the minor scales (I1-Competitive and I2-Assertive), more of a difference emerged for the Assertive scale (p < 0.001) than for the Competitive scale (p < 0.01). This indicates that, in terms of Independence, victims tended to be more submissive and non-controversial than cooperative as well as non-competitive.

In addition, a highly significant difference was found for Extroversion, with victims being less outgoing, group-oriented and more introverted than non-victims. A smaller significant difference emerged for the Conscientiousness and Social Desirability scales. Victims tended to score higher than non-victims on both scales, indicating that they were likely to be more conventional, organised, rule-bound and dependable than non-victims. For both Extroversion and Conscientiousness, similar results were seen for the minor scales.

From this initial sample it appears that victims of bullying tended to be anxious, suspicious, submissive and non-controversial, introverted, reserved, organised and conventional.

Discriminant function analysis was used to examine the ICES major scales as predictors of victim/non-victim status. The function produced had a canonical correlation with group membership of 0.89. Pooled within-group correlations between discriminating variables and the discriminant function were calculated. Stability had the highest correlation (0.86); followed by Extroversion (0.57); then Independence (0.40); and finally Conscientiousness (-0.18). Function scores correctly predicted victim/non-victim status in 96.7 per cent of the sample, with all of the victims being correctly classified as victims and 93.3 per cent of the non-victims correctly classified as non-victims. A false positive rate of 6.7 per cent and false negative rate of 0 per cent were obtained.

Results: sample 2

As for the first sample, means and standard deviations for ICES major scale sten scores were produced. A similar pattern of mean ICES sten scores between victims and non-victims was revealed by the development sample occurring within the cross-validation sample for sample 2. As before, victims were significantly lower than non-victims on Independence, Extroversion and Stability. Furthermore, they were significantly higher on the Conscientiousness scale. Although not as distant as in the first sample, the mean sten score for Stability was still at the extreme low end.

All ICES minor scales showed significant differences between victims and non-victims in the same direction as shown for major scales. Once again there was a larger difference between groups for Assertive than for Competitive scale scores. It is clear, therefore, that results from the second sample support the findings from the first sample in that victims of bullying tended to be anxious introverts who are submissive, non-controversial and conscientious.

Discriminant function analysis showed that function scores predicted correctly victim/non-victim status in 91.7 per cent of the sample, with 86.7 per cent of the victims correctly classified as victims and 96.7 per cent of non-victims correctly classified. A false positive rate of 3.3 per cent and false negative rate of 13.3 per cent were obtained.

Development of the victimisation scale

In order to test the validity of the scale robustness of the predictions, the study examined how well the function scores from sample 1 could predict sample 2 and vice versa. A double cross-validation strategy was employed. To start with, a rationally weighted composite based on the standardised canonical discriminant function coefficients of the ICES major scales in sample 1 (development sample) was produced. Integer weights were derived from the standardised canonical weights and used to construct the scale. To avoid any conceptual difficulties, the direction of the weights was then turned around so that a high score on the scale indicated victimisation – using the weights as they were would mean that a high score indicated low victimisation. From the rationally weighted composite, scale function scores for each individual were calculated. A point-biserial correlation between function scores and victim (1) and non-victim (2) status was calculated for both samples. A highly significant correlation of 0.89 (p < 0.001) was obtained for the development sample 1 (this being the canonical correlation from the discriminant function analysis) and a similar significant correlation of 0.79 (p < 0.001) for the cross-validation sample 2. In both cases victims tended to score higher on the scale than non-victims.

Secondly, a rationally weighted composite of the standardised canonical discriminant function coefficients from sample 2 was produced. As before, integer weights were derived from the standardised canonical weights, turned around, then used to construct the scale. The point-biserial correlation with victim status for the cross-validation sample 2 was 0.81 (p < 0.001), and for the development sample 1 the correlation was 0.88 (p < 0.001).

As the two rationally weighted equations developed were similar, and as strong correlations with victim status were produced from both the composite scales, a weighted composite scale was developed from the mean of the integer weights developed previously from both samples. Scale scores were then analysed via point-biserial correlations with victim status in both samples. Using the averaging criterion, point-biserial correlations with victim status were also highly significant for both sample 1 (0.89) and sample 2 (0.80). Clearly, this analysis illustrates the robustness of a weighted combination of personality traits in predicting victim status within the two samples.

Considerations arising from this study

Within workplace bullying research, there have been difficulties in obtaining an equal distribution of employees across the workplace, as most research tends to focus on white-collar employees and it is more usual that researchers have worked with victims who have contacted them – in effect, self-selecting groups. The author's clinical narrative studies are obtained under precisely these circumstances. The present study used non-self-selecting samples within two large organisations and included a wide variety of white- and blue-collar employees who represented different professions and trades. In addition, several organisational and personal criteria were matched in order to control for possible moderating effects.

The results illustrated that a control sample of non-victims in each organisation was sufficiently similar to the norm group in terms of personality to be considered representative of a working adult population, and that victims differed significantly from the control sample on all the major ICES personality scales. Victims of bullying in both organisations tended to be submissive and non-controversial, preferring to avoid conflict; conscientious, traditional, dependable and playful; quiet, reserved, with a preference for quiet and familiar surroundings; anxious, sensitive and having difficulty in coping effectively. These findings are consistent with previous research in schools (Byrne, 1994; Mynard and Joseph, 1997; Slee and Rigby, 1993) and workplaces (Einarsen *et al.*, 1994; O'Moore *et al.*, 1998; Vartia, 1996; Zapf, 1999).

This study identifies the potential usefulness of using the five-factor framework within workplace bullying research. Results from the discriminant function analysis provide some indication that a weighted composite personality profile based on the big five factors can be a robust predictor of victim status. Certainly, in the current study the weighted composite from one sample strongly correlated with victim status on the other sample. Theoretically, potential targets of bullying can be identified before they become actual victims. The moral and legal dilemmas this possibility presents are beyond the scope of this book.

The possibility, however, of being able to predict potential victim targets from personality dimensions assumes that the personality of individuals leads them to be bullied. As previously stated, Leymann (1996) strongly criticises this notion, suggesting that personality characteristics may develop more as a result of being bullied rather than being precursors to bullying. By selecting potential targets out, all that an organisation will be doing is isolating those people who have already been victims of bullying and therefore punishing them twice. However, trait theory implies that in order for a situation to have an effect on an individual (such as being bullied) the individual must have a disposition that is responsive to that effect. Stated baldly, by suffering the effects of anxiety and social withdrawal after bullying, the victim must have a disposition to be anxious and introverted rather than some other response. The material findings from developmental history (see Chapter 6) suggest strongly that this is the case.

By using the five factors as a structured framework the content of a victim personality profile is supported. The profile identified allows more of an understanding as to why personality plays a role in causing bullying at work. As suggested already by Einarsen (1999) and Zapf (1999), the perpetrators may spot weaknesses within victims' personality profiles that makes them become easy targets who are vulnerable to bullying. In relation to this study, the victims may be targeted because they are submissive and tend to avoid conflict, and hence are less likely to stand up to the perpetrators and/or less likely to develop behaviours to avoid conflict. They are highly traditional, rigid and moralistic and follow organisational norms rather than informal group norms that are contrary to formal rules; hence they may become isolated. They prefer their own company, tending to be less group-oriented and thus unlikely to have a social network to support them and deter perpetrators. In addition, they are unable to cope effectively, so the perpetrator is likely to receive positive reinforcement for acting in such a way; it is most unlikely that bullying would occur to the same extent if targets shrugged off the behaviour. Overall, by selecting these individuals, the bullies are likely to avoid retribution for their behaviour; the targets are unlikely to be able to defend themselves. In addition, due to a probable lack of social support, disapproval of the perpetrators' actions from others is unlikely to occur, as indicated by Hodges and Perry (1999) and Randall (1994) who present this argument for bullying within a school context.

The second argument relates to the notion of the 'provocative' victim (Olweus, 1993). In this case an individual's personality profile provokes aggression in others and he/she becomes the target of bullying behaviours. Zapf (as cited in Einarsen, 1999) suggests that those individuals who perceive themselves as more accurate, honest and punctual than colleagues may be thought of as patronising. Some support for this arises from the difference between groups on the Conscientious scale. Victims tended to score high on this scale and hence are generally rule-bound and moralistic (honest and punctual) as well as organised (accurate). This rigid, traditional, often perfectionistic style may annoy fellow work colleagues and lead to the individual being bullied. Also, Zapf (1999) reports that anxious behaviour (low Stability on the ICES scale) may produce a negative reaction in a group and lead to bullying. One important issue that stems from this discussion is that personality traits of victims that promote anger may be different from those traits that are vulnerable to bullying and this could relate closely to the type of bullying experienced (Einarsen, 1999). Arguably, predatory bullying of an innocent target would be experienced more by those individuals who have a personality profile that makes them vulnerable to bullies and who are targeted because of 'weaknesses' in their personality. On the other hand, the provocative victim would induce dispute-related bullying. They may not be vulnerable as such, but their traits could stimulate the bullying. A further possibility exists that the provocative victim is one who has personality traits associated with the production of complex and/or covert aggressive behaviour as well as traits of vulnerability. These may be bully–victims: those who seek to harm others by word or deed who are then subjected to dispute-related bullying.

Clinical studies of bully–victims support this last hypothesis. For example, work in progress by Coyne, Seigne and Randall using the Interpersonal

Behaviour Survey is obtaining results which differentiate adult victims from adult bully–victims. Three scales in particular form the basis of differentiation on this psychometric schedule. Whereas both groups show low scores on traits of direct aggressiveness, the bully–victims show very high scores on a scale tapping passive aggression. This is associated with complaining, negativism, procrastination and stubbornness. The verbal aggression scale is high also for the bully–victim group; this suggests the use of words as weapons and the denigration of others. These traits are irritating to co-workers who have to bear the brunt of them.

Conversely, the Conflict Avoidance scale tends to show significantly low scores; this is indicative of people who fail to recognise and avoid potential conflict and may provoke it. In common with the victim group, the bully–victim tends to show suppression on the scales associated with assertiveness but considerable elevation on the Dependency scale. This is indicative of a higher-than-average need for support and lower skills of pro-social assertion.

APPENDIX: DESCRIPTION OF ICES SCALES

'PREVUE Assessment Annex E-1: PREVUE Interpretive Manual, p. E-1:5'

Personality scales – ICES

Independent (I)

A high score (sten 8–9–10) on the Independence scale indicates a respondent who is very independent, single-minded and determined to win. They are likely to be assertive, forthright and confident. A person with this score will tend to be very sceptical and hard-headed, and may find other people's lack of drive irritating. They are good at getting things done, but can be very insensitive to the needs of those around them. They do not make good 'team players', but can be effective – though autocratic – leaders in the right circumstances.

A middle-of-the-range score (sten 4–5–6–7) would indicate a balance between a desire to compete and win and a wish to collaborate with others. Individuals like this are good at getting things done while respecting the needs of those around them. They are capable of getting their own way, although typically they are considerate and cooperative people.

Individuals with low scores (sten 1–2–3) on the Independence scale are generally likeable, diplomatic and good-natured. They are considerate and cooperative people who are capable of pulling others together. They accomplish this by encouraging and persuading others, rather than forcefully asserting their own views. An individual with a low score in Independence may skirt important issues to avoid conflict. At the extreme they are very cooperative, non-competitive, compassionate, careful of relationships and sensitive to the feelings of others. While they provide good support in a team, they may lack the assertiveness and confidence needed to pull people together and provide leadership.

The Independence scale is divided into two minor scales: Competitive and Assertive.

Competitive (11)

People who score highly (sten 8–9–10) on this scale tend to be extremely single-minded and competitive people who play to win and are bad losers. They tend to strive hard to reach their goals, putting their own success first. In playing to win, they tend to show relatively little concern about whether other people get upset or hurt along the way. In the extreme, other people are used as the means to help the person achieve their own ends.

A middle score (sten 4–5–6–7) on this scale indicates a person with a balanced mix of competitiveness and the desire to foster team spirit and work with others. Such individuals will compromise between their own need for achievement and their need to maintain cooperative relationships with others.

Those with a low score (sten 1–2–3) on this scale will be cooperative and non-competitive people who obtain their satisfaction from contributing to collaborative efforts. They are team players and enjoy cooperative ventures and are unlikely to be concerned about winning or losing. Such individuals concern themselves with maintaining personal relationships, forgoing their own success to help others, and they derive a great deal of satisfaction from the success of their team.

Assertive (12)

The high Assertiveness score (sten 8–9–10) indicates a rational, assertive and outspoken person. They know their own mind and are not afraid to say so. Individuals like this often become group leaders and are often controversial, unafraid of argument or open debate, and they will make sure their opinions are known. They will stand up for their position, even if it is unpopular or likely to create conflict.

In the middle range (sten 4–5–6–7), individuals may be fairly assertive and outspoken in some situations and with some people. They are more likely to show their assertiveness in non-threatening situations, with people they know. They tend not to promote themselves as group leaders, but with some encouragement can assume most roles. They see themselves more as peacemakers than decision makers and may appear somewhat reserved at times – being reluctant to speak out on issues.

The low scorers (sten 1–2–3) on this scale are valued for their diplomacy and tact, and can play a useful role as peacemakers and diffusers of aggression or conflict. Occasionally, they may stand up for what they see as rightly their own, but for the most part they will be a rather submissive and non-controversial person, trying to avoid conflict rather than confront it.

Conscientious (C)

A high score (sten 8–9–10) on the Conscientious scale (the C in ICES) indicates a respondent who is extremely conscientious, neat and tidy, and detail-conscious. This individual is careful to abide by the rules and is most comfortable working within clear guidelines to a set of well-defined values. They tend to hold to traditional moral values and not to be radical or innovative. People of this type are very dependable, and often meticulous in their attention to detail. Preferring to be well prepared and playful, they are likely to be good adaptors, rather than innovators.

Those in the middle range (sten 4–5–6–7) are reasonably tidy and detail-conscious in their work habits and are generally dependable, well-prepared and playful. They are comfortable with following rules and established procedures within a traditional setting. However, they are also able to work outside clear guidelines, being able to balance the need to do things well in the quickest possible way without 'breaking the rules'. This leads to solutions that may be innovative without implementing radical changes. Individuals like this are occasionally careless and disorganised, and they may need to be reminded of the framework in which they are operating.

The low scorer (sten 1–2–3) is often a spontaneous and innovative individual, who works well in changing situations. They are flexible and responsive to circumstances as they arise, and will produce creative and unorthodox solutions. You can expect some measure of chaos in their work habits as a consequence of the creativity and flexibility this individual brings to the job. While spontaneous, innovative and flexible, they will have little regard for the traditional ways of doing things. In fact, they will thrive in a creative, challenging situation, but may be unsuccessful in a highly structured and predictable environment. Individuals like this can be careless and not very well organised. If not channelled appropriately, their lack of conscientiousness can result in counter-productive behaviour.

The Conscientious scale is divided into two minor scales: Conventional and Organised.

Conventional (C1)

As a follower of the rules, a person with a high score (sten 8–9–10) on this scale will conduct themselves in a very conventional, meticulous and reliable manner. They will prefer to do things in a traditional fashion and will operate to a high moral code. Matters of principle and doing things 'the right way' are seen by such people as being of prime importance. As such, they can find it difficult to adapt to new situations or new ways of working. They are at their best working in a highly structured, clear and unambiguous environment.

The mid-range (sten 4–5–6–7) includes individuals who are reasonably conventional in their approach and their attitudes and values, and who have a balanced approach to change and innovation. These people can be flexible when necessary and can cope with change. Overall, though, they are likely to prefer the 'status quo' to change for change's sake.

Those scoring in the low range (sten 1–2–3) regard themselves as innovative and flexible, with a rather casual attitude towards guidelines, rules and regulations. They are likely to seek new ways to solve problems rather than follow traditional methods, and are likely to enjoy change for its own sake. They operate best in fast-moving and unpredictable work environments. Seeing new ways of doing things, these individuals often reach solutions by cutting corners and overlooking rules. Excelling in an ever-changing and challenging environment, they will feel stifled in a highly structured and rule-bound work situation. The possible down-side of this innovative approach is the risk of boredom or counter-productive behaviour in over-structured work situations.

Organised (C 2)

A person who scores highly (sten 8–9–10) on this is orderly and meticulous and works well in a controlled and rational environment. They have a place for everything with everything in its place. They plan ahead and think through all the possibilities before acting. They do not like having to think on their feet or engage in unstructured verbal debate. Individuals like this are often intolerant of and irritated by others who do not share these qualities. They are dependable and predictable, and find it hard to cope in situations for which they have not had a chance to prepare.

In the middle range (sten 4–5–6–7), individuals are reasonably well organised and able to work in a controlled manner. However, they do show spontaneity and are able to respond well to unpredictable events. They are reasonably neat and tidy in their working habits without being overly fastidious. While they probably do plan ahead, they do not feel particularly uncomfortable if they have to change their plans at the last minute.

Low scorers (sten 1–2–3) on this scale regard themselves as creative, spontaneous people who prefer to react to situations as they arise rather than to plan things in advance. They like to focus on the overall picture rather than deal with the fine details and do not like to worry about the details of how things will get done. Individuals like this feel that planning and structure restrict their creative and innovative abilities. They see attention to detail as being something for other people to worry about. This can manifest itself in a disorganised workplace and a failure to meet deadlines and turn up for appointments.

Extrovert (E)

Those who score highly (sten 8–9–10) on the Extrovert scale (the E in ICES) are sociable and talkative individuals who often seek excitement. These people are happiest when they are the centre of attention, seeking out people for fun, entertainment, company and stimulation. Others may see them as high-spirited, popular, 'fun' people who often act on impulse.

Individuals who score in the middle range (sten 4 5–6–7) show moderate levels of extroversion. They are generally enthusiastic and lively, contributing to social interaction without drawing undue attention to themselves. They enjoy being with others and also enjoy their own company: they have a balance between the need for companionship and the need to have time for oneself.

The low scorer (sten 1–2–3) is introverted and prefers to avoid large social gatherings and group activities. Such people are most comfortable in a quiet environment where the surroundings are familiar. They are quite content to be alone, where they can reflect on their own thoughts and ideas. They much prefer the company of a few close friends to large gatherings of acquaintances.

The Extrovert scale is divided into two minor scales: Group-oriented and Outgoing.

Group-oriented (E I)

High scorers (sten 8–9–10) on this scale have a strong need for other people. They like to be with other people and need their approval and support. They are happiest working in situations where there is a reasonable amount of contact with others and want to be seen as part of the team. They are likely to be very upset by social disapproval. Because of their need for other people, they may appear to be very sociable and they seek out environments where they can meet lots of people. While they may prefer to be with other people rather than on their own, they are not necessarily particularly outgoing. They like to be part of the group, but not necessarily the leader or the most outspoken member.

Those in the average range (sten 4–5–6–7) enjoy the company of others and may seek others out, but do not need to be with other people all the time. They like to have some time to reflect and enjoy their own company. These needs are fairly evenly balanced. In general, such people will be happiest working in situations where there is a moderate amount of contact with other people and will cope well with any need for people to collaborate and work together.

Individuals who score in the low range (sten 1–2–3) of this scale are happy to work on their own and in quiet places, and tend to avoid noisy situations and group activities. They will often avoid social gatherings, group activities and busy environments. Individuals like this are generally to be found away from the social scene and feel most at ease in their own company where they can reflect on their own thoughts, and control the amount of stimulation that reaches them. They are well-adapted to work situations where they might have to spend prolonged periods of time without direct contact with other people. While they can work with others, they do not feel any great need to.

Outgoing (E 2)

High scorers (sten 1–2–3) on this scale will be outgoing and talkative. They want to be the centre of attention. Such people enjoy 'risky', action-packed and challenging lives. They often act impulsively, and like meeting new people and doing exciting and stimulating things. Routine work may become boring for them, and they often find stimulating change in their work by moving jobs more often than others. They tend to like people for the stimulation they provide rather than need people for the support they can give (compared with E1).

Those in the average range (stens 4–5–6–7) like to lead a moderately exciting life and may act on impulse at times. They are fairly talkative and outgoing. While they find routine tasks tolerable, they would prefer some variety in their work. These people like to choose the situations in which they will take centre stage, as they are comfortable in the company of others, but they do not seek constant attention from others.

The low scorers (sten 1–2–3) describe themselves as people who are quiet and reserved, feeling that life is mentally stimulating enough without seeking extra exciting activities. Such people are not as readily bored by repetitive work and, while they may act impulsively at times, they prefer to live a quiet, orderly life. They do not like being the centre of attention, and may therefore keep in the background at social gatherings – or avoid them altogether.

Stable (S)

A score in the high range (sten 8–9–10) of this scale would indicate a stable and untroubled person, who is able to accept people at face value. For the most part, they have a relaxed approach to life, taking problems, people and circumstances in their stride. They may occasionally become anxious or suspicious, but that is the exception for them. When under normal levels of pressure or stress at work, they will remain relaxed and secure. The person high on Stability can accept criticism without feeling threatened by it and is untroubled by setbacks. As people, they are very secure in themselves and emotionally 'hardy', being able to remain calm and relaxed even when under considerable stress.

In most situations, people who score in the middle range (sten 4–5–6–7) on this scale are able to accept and deal with situations in a calm and stable manner. There will be some circumstances where they become rather apprehensive and emotional, and they may at times be wary about other people, particularly about their motives. In general, such people are reasonably secure in themselves, remaining fairly relaxed under moderate levels of stress.

A low score (sten 1–2–3) indicates someone who can be rather anxious. They tend to be suspicious of new people and wary of new situations. Sensitive and emotional, they appear to experience feelings of guilt and sadness more readily and openly than others. When faced with adversity, setbacks and other stressful situations, these people can become anxious and irritable and may find it difficult to cope effectively.

The Stable scale is divided into two minor scales: Poised and Relaxed.

Poised (S 1)

People with a high score (sten 8–9–10) on this scale readily shrug off criticism. They are able to cope with most situations in life without getting upset or irritated. They have a rational approach to life and accept that few things in life proceed without challenge or setback. They can cope with adversity without 'losing their cool'.

People with a medium score (sten 4–5–6–7) have an average balance between calm objectivity in the face of difficult situations and a tendency to be upset and take things personally at times. In some circumstances, they have difficulty being objective and rational about situations in which they are personally involved.

Those with low scores (sten 1–2–3) can be irritable and are easily upset, often losing their temper. However, their irritation and upset are usually short-lived. Individuals with such an outlook often view the world as basically hostile and threatening, and may feel that people who do not see it this way are unreasonable or naive. They find it hard to cope with embarrassing situations, and have difficulty coping with setbacks and personal criticism.

Relaxed (S 2)

A high score (sten 8–9–10) indicates a person who is very relaxed, untroubled and well prepared to cope with life's pressures. They will accept people at face value, without suspecting them of ulterior motives. People like this can leave job-related troubles and worries behind them when they go home, and they usually sleep well. They are not unduly bothered when things go wrong. However, their calm acceptance of life and their trust in the people around them may put them at risk of being exploited by others in some situations.

They can cope well with demanding high-pressure jobs, and jobs where there is a need to work with others in an open and trusting manner.

A medium score (sten 4–5–6–7) indicates a person who remains calm and relaxed in response to most situations. For the most part, individuals like this are able to manage their problems without undue anxiety. Such individuals will not always assume the best of other people, and will feel the need to check their motives at times. They tend to worry and become somewhat anxious at times, particularly when things do not go well. However, both their level of suspicion of others and their stress under pressure are likely to be moderate and not cause any difficulties.

A person with a low score (sten 1–2–3) on this scale is likely to be a rather excitable and anxious person who is rather wary and cautious of others. Individuals like this find it difficult to cope with high levels of pressure without becoming tense and anxious. They tend to be very suspicious of others whom they do not know well and may also feel that colleagues are not to be trusted. If taken to extremes, this can cause problems in interpersonal situations. Individuals like this are best-advised to avoid work situations in which there are likely to be prolonged periods of high pressure, or where they are expected to work with others in a very open and trusting manner.

Social Desirability (SocDes)

A high score (sten 8–9–10) on this scale may indicate a person who is not being totally frank in their assessment. They may be presenting what they feel to be a socially acceptable view of themselves rather than an honest picture of how they really are. Scores on other scales, particularly Conscientiousness and Stability, can be significantly influenced by this tendency. These individuals will be very certain of what is expected of them and what is proper in social situations. However, a high SocDes score can also be obtained by someone who is being honest, and who is a genuinely 'good' person. Thus a high score (particularly 9 or 10) should be regarded as an indicator of a possible distorted profile – and not taken as proof of it.

A medium score (sten 4–5–6–7) on this scale indicates a person who has presented a reasonably frank picture of themselves on the other scales.

A low score (sten 1–2–3) on Social Desirability can have two interpretations. Either the person has presented a negative impression of themselves or they have presented a frank picture of themselves but are rather lacking in a number of socially desirable attributes. In either case, the meaning of a low score would need to be explored with the person.

Part 4

Assessment outcomes and clinical consequences

Chapter 8

The effects of adult bullying

The major effects of long-term and severe bullying are outlined in Chapter 1. From that overview it may be seen that these effects are several and multi-dimensional. The effects are not straightforward, particularly on mental health, and, as will be described, span at least three major varieties of psychiatric illnesses. Post-traumatic stress disorder (PTSD), social anxiety disorder and depression are all well represented amongst the victims of workplace bullying, although it is the first of these that is most subject to research. Many anti-bullying protagonists have seized on to these serious mental health issues to demonstrate how badly treated many victims are, but they often forget that many victims have a history of mental health problems which are exacerbated rather than caused by the bullying.

Perhaps the simplest direct effects of bullying are to be found in its impact on physical health although the mechanisms are generally psychosomatic. Thus, psychosomatic stress symptoms such as muscular pain, tension, headaches, gastric upsets and elevated blood pressure are amongst the most common. Often, however, these physical symptoms are closely associated with the onset of mental health difficulties. Einarsen and Raknes (1991, cited in Hoel, Rayner and Cooper, 1999) reported on musculo-skeletal symptoms, and a year later Leymann (1992) wrote about psychosomatic stress symptoms. He also determined that there were cognitive dysfunctions in relation to concentration and emotional lability accompanying gastric upsets and nausea. These accounted for the greatest differences between the bullied and the non-bullied populations. The Einarsen and Raknes study found that the musculo-skeletal symptoms were associated with depression and a psychological strain which is manifested as anxiety and nervous lability. Hoel, Rayner and Cooper (1999) reported that bullying frequently causes psychological difficulties of depression, anxiety and nervousness attendant upon psychosomatic symptoms and cognitive effects such as attentional dysfunction, lack of initiative, irritability and insecurity.

Some researchers have reported that women show a higher presentation of somatic problems, musculo-skeletal strain and depression than men (e.g. Zapf, Knotz and Kulla, 1996). Researchers suggest that this difference may in part be explained by the fact that women are generally over-represented amongst people with psychological difficulties. The relationship between aggressive treatment and stress is well demonstrated by research. Child abuse, for example, is associated with post-traumatic stress (e.g. Famularo, Fenton and Kinscherff, 1993) which is also linked with bullying in schools (e.g. Olafsen and Viemero, 2000) and domestic violence (e.g. Linares, Groves, Greenberg, Bronfman, Augustyn and Zuckerman, 1999). A research study of workplace bullying amongst university employees also reported the experience of symptoms similar to PTSD (Bjorkqvist, Osterman and Hjelt-bäck, 1994), and single subject reports (e.g. Weaver, 2000) on bullied individuals are consistent in finding PTSD or variants upon it.

Many authors claim that exposure to bullying in adulthood is likely to be associated with negative behavioural patterns (e.g. Field, 1997). Various reports by unions and the CBI make much of increased sickness, absenteeism and leaving employment but little has been done to demonstrate cause and effect. Whereas it seems obvious that some of the victims of bullying may seek to escape their torment by remaining away from work, others may feel that they have to minimise assertions that they are not capable of working effectively by struggling on (Field, 1997). Either way, productivity is likely to be affected because, even for those victims who do not take sick leave or leave the organisation, their performance is affected by reductions in initiative, motivation and creativity (Bassman, 1992). Suicidal ideation is probably another fairly frequent effect of bullying, as indicated by a substantial number of victims who have reported such thoughts to the author. This clinical experience is supported by research studies. For example, Rigby and Slee (1999b) reported that adolescent students who are frequently victimised at school by their peers and feel generally unsupported when they have problems, are, in general, more likely to report suicidal ideation than others. This is hardly surprising because, once psychiatric illness is controlled for, elevated suicide risk is associated with adolescent psychosocial problems, particularly at school (e.g. Gould, Fisher, Parides, Flory and Shaffer, 1996).

The relationship between bullying and post-traumatic stress disorder (PTSD) has been thoroughly researched by many people. Before their work is reviewed it is perhaps helpful to consider the diagnostic criteria of PTSD as given in the diagnostic and statistical manual of mental disorders provided by the American Psychiatric Association (DSM-IV, APA, 1994).

A   The person has been exposed to a traumatic event in which both the following were present:

  (1) the person experienced, witnessed or was confronted with an event or events that involved actual or threatened death or serious injury, or a threat to the physical integrity of self or others.
  (2) the person's response involved intense fear, helplessness, or horror.

B   The traumatic event is persistently re-experienced in one or more of the following ways:

(1) recurrent and intrusive distressing recollections of the event, including images, thoughts, or perceptions.
(2) recurrent distressing dreams of the event.
(3) acting or feeling as if the traumatic event were recurring (includes a sense of reliving the experience, illusions, hallucinations, and dissociative flashback episodes, including those that occur on awakening or when intoxicated).
(4) intense psychological distress at exposure to internal or external cues that symbolise or resemble an aspect of the traumatic event.
(5) physiological reactivity on exposure to internal or external cues that symbolise or resemble an aspect of the traumatic event.

C   Persistent avoidance of stimuli associated with the trauma and numbing of general responsiveness (not present before the trauma), as indicated by three or more of the following:

(1) efforts to avoid thoughts, feelings, or conversations associated with the trauma
(2) efforts to avoid activities, places, or people that arouse recollections of the trauma
(3) inability to recall an important aspect of the trauma
(4) markedly diminished interest or participation in significant activities
(5) feeling of detachment or estrangement from others
(6) restricted range of affect
(7) sense of a foreshortened future (e.g. does not expect to have a career, marriage, children, or a normal life span)

D   Persistent symptoms of arousal, as indicated by two or more of the following:

(1) difficulty falling asleep or staying asleep
(2) irritability or outbursts of anger
(3) difficulty concentrating
(4) hypervigilance
(5) exaggerated startle response

E   Duration of the disturbance (symptoms in Criteria B, C, and D) is more than 1 month.

F   The disturbance causes clinically significant distress or impairment in social, occupational, or other important areas of functioning.

As may be seen from these criteria, a person with severe PTSD will not be able to have even an approximation to a normal life. For many, the intrusive recollections of the trauma are so overwhelming that concentration upon other matters is impossible. In addition, the suddenness with which images of the trauma can rear up is such that many sufferers are constantly on their guard, waiting for the next assault on their thoughts and senses. Their distress is impossible to hide and as a consequence many experience profound humiliation at their 'breakdown' in public or simply in front of their families. One victim of prolonged physical and verbal bullying described his experiences of PTSD as an 'endless, waking nightmare which prevented everything I took for granted – like loving my children properly'.

Arguably, the most detailed study of the relationship between adult workplace bullying and PTSD is that reported by Leymann and Gustafsson (1996). This study concerns specifically that version of workplace bullying referred to as 'mobbing' and began with an initial sample size of 2,428 subjects. Analysis revealed that 350 of these had been subjected to mobbing, and the individuals replied to questions concerning a number of stress symptoms used by the Swedish National Board of the Occupational Health Research Institute. The individuals had to comment as to whether they had had symptoms during the last twelve months on a basis of very often (or constantly), often, less often or seldom, or never. Statistical analysis of this material led to the hypothesis that PTSD and General Anxiety Disorder would be an appropriate psychiatric diagnosis. Although the 1996 study made use of a previous version of the international classification of mental disorders (DSM-III-R), the criteria for PTSD have changed little before inclusion in the most recent version, DSM-IV.

A factor analysis of the symptom results was applied and seven factor groups were identified after rotation. Of these, the first five are the most important from the clinical perspective; these five are relatively easy to determine from either general medical or psychiatric perspectives. The first factor deals with cognitive effects associated with strong stress-evoking stimuli and producing psychological hyper-reactions. This includes memory disturbances, concentration difficulties, depression and apathy, ready irritation, general restlessness, aggressiveness, feelings of insecurity and sensitivity.

The second group suggests a syndrome with psychosomatic stress characteristics including nightmares, abdominal/stomach irritation, diarrhoea and vomiting, sensation of sickness, loss of appetite, lumpy throat, crying, and loneliness.

The third factor loads heavily on to excess activity of the autonomic nervous system. This includes chest pains, sweating, dryness of the mouth, palpitations, shortness of breath, and blood pressure variation. The fourth factor concerns symptoms that are found amongst people who have been subjected to high levels of stress for very long periods of time. This is the musculoskeletal factor on which backache, neck pain and general muscular pain load heavily. The fifth factor is also associated with individuals who have been subjected to stress over a long period and have developed sleep difficulties. The items that load most heavily on it were found to be difficulties of falling asleep, interrupted sleep and early awakening. Leymann and Gustafsson (1996) quite rightly point up the similarities between these five factors and the DSM-III-R criteria of PTSD.

The sixth and seventh factors show some similarity to PTSD and include weakness in the legs, feelings of feebleness, fainting and tremor. Leymann and Gustafsson show that factors four, six and seven suggest a 'motor tension'; factors two and three suggest 'autonomic hyperactivity'; and factors one and five suggest 'vigilance and scanning'. They point up that the constituents of these factors are indicative of 'generalised anxiety disorder'. These findings indicate that repeated experiences of mobbing are associated with the development of PTSD and generalised anxiety disorder.

Leymann and Gustafsson (1996) discuss the fact that both the international classifications of psychiatric disorder (ICD-10 and DSM-III-R) of that time, state that post-traumatic stress disorder can result in permanent personality change in its chronic phase. The authors of the study refer to individuals within their clinical experience who, after several years of endeavouring to protect themselves, still suffer from lengthy and daily victimisation at work. They suggest that their research evidence does not support the view that personality characteristics are antecedents to mobbing. They state that it is not possible to evaluate a victim's original personality structure if that person is within a chronic phase of PTSD. Instead:

> What is diagnosed is the destruction of the personality. Since PTSD-injured individuals show the same syndrome and thereby the same behaviour and symptom mix (namely the syndrome that is called PTSD), it is common that professionals who are not experienced in the diagnosis of PTSD falsely assume that it is a certain type of personality that is affected by difficulties following violent events, mobbing, being taken hostage, raped, catastrophe, etc.
>
> (Leymann and Gustafsson, 1996, p. 257)

This study does not, however, indicate that any attempt had been made to take detailed personal/social histories of these subjects and, as a consequence, is cut off from an important vein of data which could have indicated earlier psychological dysfunctions and developmental/historical antecedents to them.

Nevertheless, the study proceeds to analyse the development of mobbing-related PTSD in more detail. In order to do so, Leymann and Gustafsson study data from 64 patients at the Swedish RehabCenter Inc., Violen. This institution is a private clinic employing a specially designed treatment programme for mobbing victims displaying chronic PTSD. In general, this institution caters for clients who have experienced distressing psychological responses to psychological trauma such as being in bank robberies, industrial accidents, serious car accidents, victimisation at work and other stressors.

To some extent the absence of a personal history from the first part of the study is addressed in the second where the authors described the taking of an occupational-social anamnesis. It appears, however, that this was restricted to a chronological description of the traumatic course of events which had impacted on the subjects during the two years prior to the study. The paper does not clarify whether a full developmental history was taken in addition to the medical history.

The subjects were then presented with psychometric schedules to complete and the results of these are summarised below.

Analysis of the occupational groups spanned by the subjects showed that there was significant under- and over-representation in respect of many of the major occupational types, and there was certainly a heavy preponderance of professionals working in public administration, social work and health care; the authors nevertheless claim corresponding trends with other studies.

The length of time the individuals were subjected to stress varied considerably, but only 15 per cent of the patients had a strain period of less than one year, whereas most of the subjects, 54 per cent, had a strain period of between 2 and 8 years. Some, 15 per cent, exceeded the 8-year period. There were no significant gender differences.

Subjects took the Impact of Event Scale (Horowitz, Wilner and Alvarez, 1979) which is commonly used when patients are thought to demonstrate post-traumatic responses. The results showed that 81 per cent of the subjects experienced severely intrusive recollections and 67 per cent showed high scores in relation to avoidance. This represents strong support for an appropriate diagnosis of PTSD.

A questionnaire tapping sleep patterns and alertness from the Carolina Institute Sleep Laboratory revealed that over 60 per cent of the sample experienced significant difficulties in respect of sleep disturbance. These people showed a high frequency of difficulties commonly associated with PTSD, including difficulty in falling asleep, difficulty in awakening, restless sleep, nightmares, tiredness during the day, eye irritations, falling asleep during the day and being mentally tired during the day.

The responses to the Beck Depression Inventory (Beck, Ward, Mendelson, Mock and Erbaugh, 1961) indicated that 33 per cent of the sample had a moderate depression, whilst 39 per cent experienced depression at a level normally associated with a need for medical treatment.

The subjects were also given the Post-Traumatic Symptom Scale (PTSS-10, Raphael, Lundin and Weisaeth, 1989). This is a preliminary screening instrument; whereas it does not reveal the presence of a PTSD reaction, it does reveal the need for extensive diagnostic follow-up. More than half of the subjects scored highly on this scale. Use of the General Health Questionnaire (GHQ, Goldberg and Williams, 1988) revealed that 75 per cent of the subjects were so affected by the psychological difficulties as to experience a marked reduction in their life quality. The authors endeavoured to liken the severity of the PTSD effects experienced by the subjects to those of other individuals who had been traumatised by other stressors. It was discovered that the overall strength of the PTSD effects experienced by these subjects was greater than those experienced by train drivers who had run over and killed suicidal people on railway and subway lines. The authors consider that the trauma associated with mobbing extends beyond the actual experiences of victimisation in the workplace into the post-mobbing environment where additional difficulties are experienced with the judicial and health care systems. They state that mobbed employees suffered from a 'traumatic environment' (p. 272) where psychiatrists, insurance offices, personnel departments, managers and co-workers, trade unions, doctors, etc. can act in such a way as to produce further traumatic difficulties. The authors liken their mobbed subjects to raped women who find themselves under continuing threat: 'As long as the perpetrator is free, the woman can be attacked again. As long as the mobbed individual does not receive effective support, he or she can, at any time, be torn to pieces again' (p. 273). As a result it is inevitable that the PTSD symptoms cannot remain as the same traits as those of an individual who has experienced one-off trauma. Leymann and Gustafsson state that the extremely prolonged stress duration seriously threatens the victim's socio-economic existence: 'Torn out of their social network, a life of early retirement with permanent psychological damage threatened the greatest majority of mobbing victims' (Leymann and Gustafsson, 1996, p. 273).

The significance of long-term mobbing in terms of its effects on the individual and his/her family was made obvious by the tragic case of a 33-year-old machine operator in Yorkshire who was victimised by fellow workers when they discovered he was dyslexic and could not read. As already described, on a number of occasions his colleagues trussed him up in shrink-polythene wrapping which, on one occasion, almost suffocated him. Although he complained to the management, nothing was done to support him and eventually he left his job after eighteen months of victimisation. He was awarded a record-breaking £28,000 for injury to feelings which, at the time, was more than three times the previous highest award. The man in question reported that the level of distress he was caused and the effects on him caused severe relationship difficulties with his partner and their children.

CASE STUDY

Ryan was a 33-year-old machine operator in a plastic moulding factory. He had been in steady employment since leaving school at the age of 16 years and had mainly worked as a semi-skilled machinist. He moved to the plastic factory at the age of 31 years, having been made redundant.

Ryan described himself as a 'nervy person' and once had had treatment for stress-related facial tics and involuntary hand spasms. This had been associated with a variety of stressors including the death of his mother from cancer, a messy divorce and job insecurity. He was involved in a severe car accident which led to him being treated for anxiety and depression.

His developmental history showed anxious attachment to his parents which was associated with overprotection and 'smothering' after his mother lost her second son to a viral illness. Ryan stated that he had been bullied at primary and secondary school where his teachers thought that he was 'too much of a mother's boy and needed toughening up'. During interview Ryan revealed that he had never really recovered from the bullying at school and shared the negative evaluations held of himself by his bullies. He described himself as 'weak and indecisive, always unwilling to take a chance but terrified of criticism for doing a bad job'. He saw himself as someone who could not hold on to relationships and cited his wife leaving him as evidence.

He had felt extremely threatened at the prospect of moving to the new job because he had heard that the plastic factory was a hard environment to work in. He stated, 'I always knew I would get bullied again some day – it always surprised me that it took them [bullies] so long to get round to it.'

Ryan believed that the bullying started because he did not want to join the men in a football pools club. He was having a hard time paying maintenance at the time and was aware that the Child Support Agency was investigating his circumstances. As a result he felt he did not have money to spare for gambling. 'For some reason the men took exception to this and talked about it to the supervisor. I explained that I knew nothing about football and did not particularly like it. That was it – from then on they never left me alone.'

Ryan was subjected to mobbing involving insults, isolation, spoiling of his work output, hiding his materials, pushing, shoving and adulterating his canteen meals. He complained to the supervisor but was told that the three principal perpetrators had all worked well for the company for a long time and no one had ever complained about them before. The supervisor then called the three men into his office and required that Ryan repeat his accusations. 'I was very nervous but got through it – they just stood there – said I was talking crap and lying, then they went. The supervisor just looked at me and shrugged his shoulders.' Later that day Ryan's car was smeared with resin.

Given the passive support of the supervisor, the three men increased their efforts at mobbing and added a fourth man to the group. By this time the mobbing was a daily event of nearly eight months' duration.

Ryan began to experience a series of intense stress symptoms and took short periods of sick leave. The bullying affected his work output when he was in the factory and the supervisor warned him that he was falling below an acceptable standard.

The stress symptoms intensified and Ryan experienced severe sleep disorder, appetite loss and hypervigilance. He found he was unable to concentrate on even routine tasks or simple television programmes. His interest in gardening drained away from him and he stopped having contact with his two children.

Intrusive thoughts about the bullying were very frequent and he experienced painful 'flashbacks', mainly concerning episodes of humiliation in the canteen or other public places in the factory. By degrees, he became increasingly unable to go anywhere near the factory or the route he used to drive to it.

He was seen by a psychiatrist who diagnosed PTSD.

Social anxiety disorder

As can be seen from any review of the literature, the diagnosis of PTSD has rather dominated investigation into the major clinical effect of workplace bullying. In the writer's clinical experience, the majority of bullied workers seldom meet the full criteria for a diagnosis of post-traumatic stress disorder, but this does not mean that those symptoms of post-traumatic stress that they do experience are not distressing and debilitating. Many other victims experience a lesser-known disorder which is referred to in the international classification systems as Social Anxiety Disorder or, sometimes, Social Phobia. This is an extremely debilitating disorder as well and one would be hard put to state confidently which was the worse from the viewpoint of victims.

The clearest diagnostic criteria for social anxiety disorder are provided by DSM-IV (APA, 1994). These criteria are as follows:

A A marked and persistent fear of one or more social or performance situations in which the person is exposed to unfamiliar people or to possible scrutiny by others. The individual fears that he or she will act in a way (or show anxiety symptoms) that will be humiliating or embarrassing. Note: In children, there must be evidence of the capacity for age-appropriate social relationships with familiar people and the anxiety must occur in peer settings, not just in interactions with adults.

B Exposure to the feared social situation almost invariably provokes anxiety, which may take the form of a situationally bound or situationally predisposed panic attack. Note: In children, the anxiety may be expressed by crying, tantrums, freezing or shrinking from social situations with familiar people.

C   The person recognises that the fear is excessive or unreasonable. Note: In children, this feature may be absent.
D   The feared social or performance situations are avoided or else are endured with intense anxiety or distress.
E   The avoidance, anxious anticipation, or distress in the feared social or performance situations(s) interferes significantly with the person's normal routine, occupational (academic) functioning, or social activities or relationships, or there is marked distress about having the phobia.
F   In individuals under the age of 18 years, the duration is at least 6 months.
G   The fear or avoidance is not due to the direct physiological effects of a substance (e.g. a drug of abuse, a medication) or a general medical condition and is not better accounted for by another mental disorder (e.g. Panic Disorder with or without Agoraphobia, Separation Anxiety Disorder, Body Dysmorphic Disorder, a Pervasive Developmental Disorder, or Schizoid Personality Disorder).
H   If a general medical condition or another mental disorder is present, the fear in Criterion A is unrelated to it, e.g. the fear is not of Stuttering, trembling in Parkinson's disease, or exhibiting abnormal eating behaviour in Anorexia Nervosa or Bulimia Nervosa.

Social anxiety disorder has only recently gathered recognition as a unique anxiety disorder distinguishable from other psychiatric disorders. Nevertheless, there remain several areas in which this distinction is not straightforward, a position that is further confused by its considerable comorbidity with other disorders which can make differentiated diagnosis problematic. For example, social anxiety disorder cannot be diagnosed where there is major depression, panic disorder with agoraphobia, generalised anxiety disorder, obsessive-compulsive disorder, and body dysmorphic disorder.

The main presenting feature for the diagnosis of social anxiety disorder is an excessive fear of being observed or scrutinised in particular performance contexts. Where individuals were simply anxious being around people they were deemed to have avoidant personality disorder and were excluded from the diagnosis of social anxiety disorder. As, however, Moutier and Stein (1999) point out, many people who met the criteria for social anxiety disorder also experienced more generalised anxiety over a wide variety of social settings. This finding led to broadening of the diagnostic criteria.

The key diagnostic feature is retained as an excessive fear of scrutiny by others, leading to familiar symptoms of anxiety such as blushing, tremulousness and palpitations. There must be a pronounced reduction in functioning and/or marked distress in order for the criteria to be confirmed. Social anxiety disorder is described as having two subtypes, generalised and non-generalised. The generalised subtype is made up of sufferers who are anxious in most performance (e.g. speaking in public, demonstrating tasks, being monitored) and interactional (e.g. conversational, public transport, shopping) situations. In the writer's experience, the majority of workplace victims tend to fall within the realms of this subtype. The non-generalised subtype is characterised by people who become highly anxious and unable to function in particular performance locations but who seem to function reasonably successfully in others (Kessler, Stein and Berglund, 1998).

The reduction in functioning can be very severe (Moutier and Stein, 1999), even to the point that affected individuals are unable to see their doctors or disguise the extent of the impact on them. Prevalence of this disorder in the US has been assessed at 13.3 per cent (Kessler, McGonagle, Zhao *et al.*, 1994), which is greater than that of major depressive and alcohol-related disorders in that country.

Social anxiety disorder has significant epidemiological findings showing consistent socio-demographic characteristics amongst individuals with the disorder. It was more common amongst women who were young, unmarried, with only basic education and of low socio-economic status. Young men with a similar profile were present in the survey but the female-to-male ratio was 3:2. Age of onset was typically between 13 and 20 years for both sexes and onset after 25 was rare.

Of significance to the study of bullying, this survey found that half of the people with the disorder did not complete high school. Clinical experience of many severely bullied adolescents indicates that they ceased attending secondary education because they were bullied and so failed to gain qualifications. Heimberg and colleagues (1990, 8.3) reported that individuals with generalised social anxiety disorder tended to be less well-educated and less likely to be employed than those with non-generalised disorder. Age of onset in adolescence is highly predictive of the disorder continuing into adulthood, and mean durations of the illness have been reported in excess of twenty years (e.g. Moutier and Stein, 1999).

The following case study is of a young woman whose condition may be differentiated clearly from PTSD and other disorders such that a diagnosis of Social Anxiety Disorder is inevitable.

CASE STUDY

Carol, aged 20 at the time of referral, was a care assistant working with elders in a local authority home. She had been in that or similar jobs since she left school at the age of 16. Carol was of low average ability and had no formal qualifications. Her GCSE results were D or below and she had required remedial assistance in respect of literacy and numeracy.

She was the youngest child of a big family with four brothers and three sisters, all of whom had low-status employment or were on income support. Her alcoholic father had sexually abused two of her sisters but left the two youngest unscathed, largely because his drinking took priority. Carol entered care work from a YTS scheme and found that she was well supported by other staff. She enjoyed the work and made numerous friends amongst the elderly residents. After one year of employment she was redeployed along with other staff with the closure of the house she was in. For a further year all went well and she continued to flourish.

One week after her eighteenth birthday and engagement party, Carol and her co-workers were told that there would be further contractions in the local authority services. The staff recognised that this would probably result in redundancies and stress levels rose. There was a view that only a certain number of the best staff could be kept on. As the area was one of high unemployment, it meant a lot that the women kept their work. Carol said later that she did not really understand the issues; her own disposition was such that she expected everything to be sorted out and so did not predict big changes taking place for her.

Gradually other staff who had been supportive of her began to become irritable with her. They resented her frequent questions and having to make allowances for her ability. They disliked also the easy familiarity she had with the residents who often gave her little treats or presents. She was subjected then to a pattern of verbal bullying and isolation. Other staff challenged her work standards and made trivial reports about her to the senior administrative officer. People refused to work with her and she was accused of dangerous practices with some of the more frail and vulnerable residents. She was slapped across the face by one member of staff who accused Carol of looking at her in a 'wicked way', and was pushed and shoved by other members of staff. Quite rapidly, Carol found that the work she loved was associated with a high level of stress.

On numerous occasions Carol's work was publicly criticised by other staff. This occurred in front of residents and supervisory staff. The only note taken by the employment officer was a 'Be careful with that lot; they're bad news.'

Carol's mental health deteriorated as the bullying persisted and increased in intensity. Soon she began to try to avoid shifts that the worst of the bullies shared with her. This was not entirely satisfactory because the shift pattern changed a lot. She then began to stay away from work, claiming to have minor illnesses. Eventually she stopped going altogether, even though, at that time, she was still able to move around the community without problems. Eventually, however, even that became too hard for her and she began to restrict her movements out of her home such that she went only the short distance to visit her maternal grandmother and to some very local shops. Her relationships at home continued to be largely unaffected. This was not the case on those few occasions that she was persuaded to go to work where she experienced three panic attacks, one so severe that it was thought that she was developing a form of epilepsy. By the time of her nineteenth birthday she was not going to work at all and she was unable to travel out much unless her mother was present. Her engagement had been called off. Psychiatric referral resulted in a diagnosis of social anxiety disorder for which she received medication. Employment matters reached an impasse when she refused to go to the home to discuss her future with the employers and union representative and they refused to see her at home. Carol stated repeatedly that she could not return to a place where she was thought to be useless and disliked by so many people.

As can be seen, the fear of severe negative evaluation by others and the consequences is at the heart of this young woman's difficulties. This fear is at the core of social anxiety disorder and, perhaps because it leads the sufferer to invalidate any effort he or she can make alone, remission rarely occurs without therapeutic intervention. It is typical, as in the case above, that depression increases the burden of the disorder on the sufferer. Lépine and Pélissolo (2000) state that the socio-economic impact of social anxiety disorder is considerable on both the sufferers and the community. It is obvious that the quality of life is greatly reduced; work, community, family, social and other functioning are badly affected and many sufferers find themselves unable to move anywhere other than in a very small routinised way in a particular location. In the author's clinical experience, most young sufferers are unable to work and some are so badly affected that they are unable to attend clinic settings for therapeutic involvement. Where their condition is a result of persistent negative evaluation brought on by workplace bullying it is often nearly impossible to get them to attend meetings with employers and union representatives within the workplace and they are perceived incorrectly to be uncooperative and 'unwilling to meet us half-way'.

Carol's age of onset was fairly typical of the general pattern; late adolescence is the norm. Although the symptoms can be unremittingly durable, comorbid conditions invariably emerge. Thus Lépine and Pélissolo (2000) describe studies showing comorbid depression in 71 per cent, drug abuse and alcohol abuse in 85 per cent, and obsessive-compulsive disorder in 61 per cent of subjects.

They also describe the complexity of the relationship between social anxiety disorder and alcoholism. Sufferers may well turn to alcohol to help them deal with feelings of anxiety in social situations; excessive consumption may precipitate symptoms of anxiety (e.g. Schuckit and Hesselbrock, 1994). This link to alcoholism and other disorders creates long-term problems for individuals whose quality of life may be badly impaired for years unless treatment is provided.

Despite the obvious relationship between workplace bullying and the onset of this disorder, particularly amongst young workers, it is rare to find a diagnosis of social anxiety disorder being made even within occupational health settings. This particular trend is mirrored across primary care medical settings where it seems that social phobia is either under-diagnosed or confused with more general anxiety conditions (Stein, McQuaid, Laffaye and McCahill, 1999). Unlike severe PTSD, however, it is not clear that social anxiety disorder has the same permanent impact on personality structure. It is relatively susceptible to medication and there is considerable research evidence on the effectiveness of, for example, Paroxetine (e.g. Allgulander, 1999). Of more psychological benefit to workplace victims who have developed this disorder is the finding that cognitive-behavioural therapy may bring about positive change either alone or in combination with medication. Successful interventions of this sort are associated with acute improvements and long-term maintenance of treatment gain; typically the therapy emphasises cognitive-restructuring and exposure interventions whether within individual or group formats (Otto, 1999).

In the author's clinical experience, where social anxiety disorder is the product of workplace bullying, the victims have every reason to be fearful of a negative evaluation of themselves by others because most forms of bullying represent a severe attack on self. The problem for the sufferer is, however, that this fear of continued negative evaluation persists long after the original causes have been dealt with. It is not uncommon for such fears to persist at a psychopathological level five years or more after the bullying has ceased. Under these circumstances, it is inevitable that medication alone will not be adequate to bring about a long-term and maintained benefit. The sufferers must be helped to achieve not only a resistance to the fear but a restructuring of their own self-concept. As a consequence, estimation of the quantum of damage owed to a victim of workplace bullying with social anxiety disorder would not be complete without a calculation of the cost of individual psychotherapy, and should not be calculated on the basis of medication alone.

Body dysmorphic disorder

The author has come across several cases of this disorder or partial disorder in the context of female workers who have been subjected to a relentless tirade about their physical characteristics. Not surprisingly, the issue of body weight figures largely in this tragic situation but there are usually other aspects of the bullying which cause the victim to experience extreme dissatisfaction with their physical appearance.

People with body dysmorphic disorder (BDD) are extremely anxious about a particular aspect of their appearance. Some are concerned that their skin is pockmarked or scarred, that their hair is too thin, their nose is too big or some part is too fat. They are unable to believe family members and friends who seek to reassure them, but pay attention to others who they think are critical of their appearance. Obviously, if someone makes repeated references to some aspect of their appearance then they feel even more anxious. Often when trying to describe the particular flaw they imagine or exaggerate the sufferer tries hard not to draw attention to it and speaks only of their general ugliness.

Most individuals describe this disorder as causing them marked distress and they become so preoccupied by it that important aspects of their personal-social life are affected severely. Many spend hours each day thinking about their defect, to the point where they come to believe that they are too ugly to be seen in the community or workplace. The quality of their life is greatly affected and one recent survey (Phillips, 2000) found that the effect was greater than that for depression, diabetes or heart disorder.

It is probable that certain people are more prone to BDD than others. Phillips and McElroy (2000) showed that BDD sufferers had a significant risk elevation for personality disorders, with avoidant personality disorder being the most common; they showed also high scores on neuroticism scales and lower scores on extroversion, which are consistent with that personality disorder. Castle and Morkell (2000) reported a high comorbidity incidence with depression, social phobia and obsessive-compulsive disorder; this review indicated successful treatment possibilities from a combination of seratonergic antidepressants and cognitive-behavioural therapy. Jolanta and Tomasz (2000) reported strong links between BDD and eating disorders.

The diagnostic criteria for body dysmorphic disorder are as follows:

A   Preoccupation with an imagined defect in appearance. If a slight physical anomaly is present, the person's concern is markedly excessive.
B   The preoccupation causes clinically significant distress or impairment in social, occupational, or other important areas of functioning.
C   The preoccupation is not better accounted for by another mental disorder (e.g. dissatisfaction with body shape and size in Anorexia Nervosa).

These seemingly simple criteria disguise some related behaviours which can be of devastating intensity. Many people with BDD are found to compare their appearance frequently with that of others of the same gender and approximate age (or younger). They may be 'caught' scrutinising the appearance of people, who may react negatively to being stared at. Most will spend inordinate periods of time changing their appearance in mirrors and reflecting surfaces such as shop windows, metal panels, and pools of water. They may spend hours trying to disperse the perceived flaws and many seek plastic surgery and other medical treatments. Others go to great lengths not to see their reflection. Their friends and family become irritated by them as they constantly seek reassurance about their appearance.

Not surprisingly, many BDD sufferers engage in a variety of strategies to rid themselves of the anxiety. These involve excessive dieting and/or exercising, using drugs to build muscle and reduce fat, picking skin to remove imperfections from it, and avoiding social situations. The sad situation of a 23-year-old woman was reported in the UK press in 2000. She hardly left her parents' home and had never had a boyfriend, gone to a dance or engaged in other activities enjoyed by young people. She had been diagnosed with BDD which was said to have been caused by prolonged bullying at secondary school. This had taken the form of verbal assaults centred on her appearance. The picture of her was of an attractive young woman who had no reason to believe she was ugly. The next case study reveals a link between workplace bullying, race and BDD.

CASE STUDY

At 26, Justine, whose parents were from Taiwan, was pleased to be a legal secretary working for a big partnership with a large typing pool. She had been in the job for nearly a year after having had nearly two years away from work following a nervous breakdown. This had been stress-related and one of a series of similar difficulties that she had had from adolescence onwards. There seemed to be no particular cause; she just seemed to be susceptible to stress, as had her mother before her.

Justine had never experienced bullying at work before, although she had been a victim throughout the last two years of her primary education. Problems began when another secretary seemed to become jealous of Justine's developing friendship with one of the young solicitors. At first Justine was only aware of some of the rather personal questions: 'Aren't you a bit worried going out to posh places with him?' These became more pointed: 'He needs to go out with a really glamorous solicitor from Bradford'; and eventually very hurtful: 'Does he ever comment that your eyes look slitted?'

Justine had never had any comments passed about her ethnic background and appearance. She had never thought twice about her racial origins and this had not been an issue when she had been bullied at school. The jealous colleague noted that Justine was distressed by mention of her eyes and made more comments, spreading these out into the typing pool. Most people ignored her and some were dismissive but a few took up the theme and began to refer to Justine in similar terms.

Even after the young male solicitor left the firm and the relationship with Justine ended, the tirade of verbal aggravation continued. It had become part of the group habitual behaviour which was sustained only by the reinforcement of Justine's obvious distress. Justine became pre-occupied with the appearance of her eyes and spent increasing time in front of a mirror looking at them. She visited her GP saying that she needed corrective surgery, and would not accept the doctor's refusal on the grounds that there was nothing wrong and that she was a perfectly attractive person.

The intervention of the senior administrator stopped the tirade inside the office but this did not prevent the abuse carrying on in the office block, cafeteria and outside the building. The aggressors also made gestures at Justine, pulling at the corners of their own eyes to mime their previous insults. Justine began to feel that she was inordin-ately ugly and begged her doctor for corrective surgery. She missed days at work because she felt so stressed, and told her father that she was too ugly to be seen in a busy law firm's office. She sought help from a Eurasian counsellor, not for therapy, but simply to keep checking that her eyes were not unusual. Eventually she stopped going to work and gradually became more hesitant to go out at all. She handed in her notice and became long-term unemployed. Referral to a clinical psychologist resulted in recommendations for combined medication and cognitive therapy but she refused on the grounds that the therapist would only have to look at her face to realise how ugly she was.

Effects on family

Not surprisingly, severe disorders have a considerable impact on the families of the sufferers. The majority of the author's clients who have such diagnoses portray sad pictures of family fragmentation and dissolution as a con-sequence of their presenting symptoms. The following example is of a young woman with social anxiety disorder who lost her husband and son as a consequence of her inability to progress.

CASE STUDY

Julie's partner walked out on her taking their 18-month-old son, Ben, with him. He stated that she had allowed herself to reach such a low level of functioning that she was creating an impossible situation for a young child to thrive in.

Julie was 21 years old at this time and had been diagnosed with a social anxiety disorder only nine months after Ben's birth. She had returned to her work as an automotive part packer about a month after his birth and Ben was looked after by his maternal grandmother.

She had not particularly wanted to return to work but her desire to buy nice things for Ben could not be met from one income alone. Almost immediately she ran into verbal harassment from two women on the line who criticised her for returning to work so early. Their theme was that they had to work because they were single parents but she did not – she had Ben's father to support her.

The level of vitriol in these comments increased and other women became involved, albeit on the periphery. The increase occurred because it was rumoured that Julie's return to work resulted in the loss of work for another single mother on a temporary contract. The harassment spread out from the warehouse to the small local community from which most of the women came, including Julie. As a result the bullying extended well beyond the workplace. Eventually Julie's avoidance strategies became so extreme that she was unable to take Ben out, go to the shops and go to work. Her partner found that he had to stay off work to support her and eventually his job was threatened. Julie was diagnosed as having social phobia (social anxiety disorder) and treated accordingly.

Effects on observers

Finally, it is the case that simply being observers of bullying increases the stress levels of non-targets (Vartia, 1996). Observers can be acute observers of bullies and able to identify their characteristics. They are aware of the impact of these people as working groups and can identify what this means for work output and the general working climate (e.g. Mehta, 2000). Much work remains to be carried out to identify what kinds of observer behaviour are elicited.

Chapter 9

The report: assessment outcomes

The previous chapters have presented a framework for the assessment of critical factors in the formation of bully and victim behaviours. In this chapter the collation of assessment findings is presented for one bully and one victim. These assessments demonstrate typical findings concerning employees referred by Human Resources departments in the context of workplace bullying. Both cases reveal typical organisational and personal antecedents which fall within the model of workplace bullying presented in Chapter 2. Although not overt this structure is used to guide both assessments, and the conclusions are based on hypotheses drawn from it. Antecedents for bullying and indeed for being a victim are identified and remediation is suggested in accordance with the findings.

The first report concerns an aggressive yet insecure middle-aged line manager whose actions were impacting on more than one member of his team.

Psychological Report
on
JD (Date of Birth: 16–06–56)

Senior Admin. Officer
Payroll/Pensions Dept.
Date of Report:

1.0 *Reason for referral*
1.1 JD was referred by Human Resources because of repeated allegations of harassment and victimisation. It is alleged that he uses his size, threatening postures and abusive language to intimidate staff.
1.2 JD has been questioned by Human Resources about these allegations and has claimed that the staff concerned are poorly motivated and lazy. He states that he has needed to be firm with them in order to secure their proper output.
1.3 There are problems in his section which are evident from a higher-than-average transfer request rate. Exit rates are unacceptably high also.

2.0 *Summary*

2.1 This assessment is based upon information drawn from documentation, interviews, observations and psychometric testing. The following recommendations were made:

Whether or not the allegations of the two women are substantiated, there is a clear need to review JD's management skills.

He needs therapeutic sessions, firstly to explore these assessment findings and secondly to help him understand the need for change. To set the scene for this work it would be helpful if a senior manager could dispel his mythical thinking that his aggressive style is valued by the organisation. (If he is right, however, and his behaviour is encouraged, then the company can expect many more complaints and litigation.)

JD needs to take part in relevant people management courses and Human Resources will be able to arrange this. He then needs a period of supervision and monitoring to ensure that he does not pay lip-service to such inputs. Review in six months is vital.

3.0 *Basis of this assessment*

3.1 This assessment has made use of information from:

- the following documents

  1   Human Resources report dated _____
  2   Reports of TR and EH, accounts clerks, alleged victims
  3   Employment records
  4   JD's job description
  5   Last appraisal report

- four interview sessions with JD, each lasting one hour
- psychometric testing

4.0 *Background*

4.1 **Employment records:** JD has a series of qualifications including HNC in office systems, office management and accounts. He entered the company ten years ago with good references from a competitor. He has received one promotion and has been on three short courses concerning staff management.

4.2 There are no indications of poor relationships with other staff and he is well respected by his senior management. He has a reputation for firmness and the staff exit rate from his department is significantly above the norm.

4.3 **The complaints:** Two Administrative Officers, Ms TR and Mrs EH, allege that he has whispered obscenities at them, shouted derogatory remarks in front of colleagues and physically intimidated them by standing over them very closely. Ms TR feels particularly intimidated by his size which is probably at or beyond the 90th centile for both height and weight.

4.4 In addition, Mrs EH claims that JD has repeatedly rejected her annual leave requests, not made allowances for the death of her mother and been rude when problems of her children's health have made her late. She feels that he scrutinises her work far more closely than that of her colleagues.

4.5 Ms TR made an allegation of sexual harassment but withdrew this. She felt that the 'looming over me' that she alleges may not have been sexually motivated because she has seen JD do this to young male trainees. Nevertheless she finds it unnerving.

4.6 Both women claim that they are subject to this treatment on a daily basis. Ms TR is now on sick leave with 'anxiety and stress' on her medical certificate. This period is now of four weeks' duration and is the third sickness absence for stress-related difficulties. She alleges that this illness is the result of JD's actions and she has spoken to her union representative. She has started sessions with an external EAP counsellor and I understand that a psychiatric consultant has been arranged for her.

4.7 Mrs EH has gone off sick also and I am told that she too has a stress-related disorder.

4.8 Both women have been employees of the company for a period of years. Neither has had a significant history of ill-health absenteeism or unexplained absence. It is clear that their increased ill-health absence has arisen during the time that they allege harassment from JD.

4.9 Two co-workers have been interviewed by personnel officers and confirm some of the details of harassment provided by Mrs EH and Ms TR. They were aware of the derogatory shouted remarks and have seen JD standing very close to both women. Neither co-worker could recall hearing whispered obscenities. Neither co-worker has experienced any unfair treatment by JD but they agree that he can speak directly and firmly to make his points. One described him as 'competitive' and the other said he is 'too pushy at times'. Neither co-worker was aware of any significant reason for the alleged victims to be harassed but one had a poor opinion of Ms TR, stating that 'she is often complaining about one thing or another'.

5.0 *Interview with JD*

5.1 **Circumstances of the interview:** The first interview was held at the consulting rooms of the external EAP provider. The subsequent sessions were held at his own home where he felt less threatened.

5.2 He is a tall, well-built man who seldom smiled and who maintained an air of distance throughout. This did not stop him from being cooperative and willing to undertake the assessment. 'I'll do whatever it takes to clear my name.' He confirmed that he has no criminal convictions but has been prosecuted for speeding offences on six occasions.

5.3 JD was suspicious, however, of the psychometric testing and wanted to know if his alleged victims would also be expected to complete similar tests.

5.4 **Personal history:** JD provided a personal history during a session that was structured using the Multimodal Life History Questionnaire, which enables a detailed personal-social history to be taken.

5.5 JD agreed that 'I asserted myself strongly at school'. He had many fights but his 'assertiveness' mostly took the form of verbal threats and physical intimidation (threat of violence). He agreed that his large size made this possible for him.

5.6 He responded to a Peer Relation indicator and revealed that he did have a small group of admiring boys who assisted him when he wanted to make a point strongly. He admitted to pushing, shoving, kicking and spoiling other children's work.

5.7 He experienced several frustrations but most particularly resented that children from better-off families seemed to get better opportunities than he did. He recalled a particular child whose father was a wealthy farmer 'getting more breaks than I ever did – he needed bringing down a peg or two and people expected me to be the one to do it'. JD became quite irate as he described his school experiences and told me: 'I was even cheated out of captaining the school's senior football team by a lad who scored more goals but couldn't play as well as me.' JD felt that he was not respected by his teachers who 'only wanted to suck up to the polite kids who spent all their time swotting'.

5.8 **Attachment history:** JD's responses were analysed according to the Adult Attachment Interview. The results indicated that he experienced quite severe power-assertive methods of controlling behaviour including the occasional use of a cane by his father. He was shouted at regularly and his mother would often slap his face when she felt he was being rude or cheeky. He experienced dismissive parenting because his father did not seem to care where he was or who he was with; his mother alternated between condemning his friends and encouraging him to go to their homes so she could get on with her work as an early 'cottage industry' audio typist. As he progressed into adolescence and got a reputation for rowdy behaviour his parents clamped down on him and swung from distancing to over-controlling management. JD said 'I lived in an open prison with no remission for good behaviour.' Not surprisingly he carried these poor attachments into subsequent relationships. His marriage ended in divorce after a period of domestic violence and he soon lost contact with his son from this relationship. JD described his ex-wife as a 'female eunuch who needed to be servile but resented people stronger than her – which was nearly everybody'.

5.9 It was noteworthy, however, that he returned to a consistent theme of anxiety about abandonment. The first time this arose was in the context of his parenting. His remarks were caustic. 'I never knew if my parents loved me – my mother seemed too busy for me and I was just an irritation to my father.' The next comments were about his ex-wife: 'It wasn't a matter of if she would desert me, it was more a matter of when.' He brushed aside his own violent behaviour, saying simply that 'a saint would have hit her'. Later he expressed fears that his senior managers would 'hang me out to dry' if they became convinced by the 'stupid lies' of the complainants. Some suicidal ideas were expressed: 'what's the bloody point: I can't think of one reason for plodding on through all this shit'; 'I don't know why you're here, I've no wish to keep on going through life like this'; 'I can certainly understand why suicides bottle out, I think about it a lot – they've got it right.'

5.10 **Employment environment:** JD stated that he was aware that his senior managers appreciated the directness with which he ran the section. He alleges being complimented more than once on the way he dealt with employees who were persistently poor at time-keeping and maintained low standards of output. JD believed that his firmness was respected by his managers and also by his staff.

5.11 He reflected on increased pressures within all departments and stated: 'People aren't going to let me down – the world is getting tougher and I expect more, not less, from staff.' He spoke of the local authority restructuring that was ongoing and said: 'We've all got to watch our backs, there's too many people in the service – dead wood will get chopped out.'

5.12 Many of his comments were about 'staff'; there were few mentions of them by name. He seemed to have little idea of them as people and no interest in their personal lives and needs. His responses about his co-workers were essentially depersonalised. JD thought that his employers' policies for employees were 'wimpish' and provided 'a licence for skiving shirkers with more hang-ups than a cloakroom'.

5.13 **The allegations:** JD became angry when questioned about the alleged incidents. He left his seat and moved around the room. 'I was no firmer with them than I was with anybody. Both are always moaning and complaining; they don't seem to want to work. If I'm on their backs a lot, it's because they need it.'

5.14 He denied using obscene language in whispers and laughed angrily rather than speak of intimidatory non-verbal behaviour. He did agree, however, that he had shouted at both women 'on some rare occasions'.

5.15 He could not explore those occasions when he agreed he had shouted; he seemed unable to get beyond the 'injustice' of being 'brought to book by two slackers'. JD never reached the point where he could reflect on his behaviour or his attitudes to his co-workers; his sense of being victimised by the complainants was too strong and represented an insuperable obstacle to insight.

5.16 **Self-perceptions:** When asked to complete the 'Images' section of the Multimodal Life History Questionnaire, he indicated that 'Succeeding', 'Being aggressive', 'Being talked about' and 'Being in charge' applied to him. When asked to complete the 'Thoughts' section, he indicated that 'Intelligent', 'Confident', 'Worthwhile' and 'Hard-working' applied to him. When asked to add other words or phrases of his own, he provided 'Unforgiving' and 'Perceptive'. Unexpectedly, but congruent with his interview responses, he added also 'Self-damaging'.

6.0 *Psychometric testing*

6.1 JD was given three psychometric schedules to complete. These are the Personality Assessment Inventory (PAI), the Interpersonal Behaviour Survey (IBS) and the Firestone Self-Destructive Thoughts Test (FAST). The first of these is a self-administered objective inventory of adult personality designed to provide information on critical clinical variables. It is a modern and powerful inventory containing 344 items tapping 22 mutually exclusive scales which include 4 validity scales. The latter are sensitive detectors of people who 'fake good' or 'fake bad', respond inconsistently and/or randomly. The second schedule (IBS) is a sensitive measure of the different ways in which people respond to others in their normal community settings. Included amongst these scales are three which deal with response types associated with the conscious or unconscious distortion of interpersonal behaviour. Thus one scale deals with denial, a second with random responding and a third with impression management (Fake good). These scales are generic in that they are associated with interpersonal behaviour generally rather than in specific relation to workplace settings. The third scale (FAST) is a psychometric schedule recording suicidal ideation (thoughts about suicide, feelings of helplessness and behaviour associated with suicide attempts).

6.2 JD was found to have significant scores on a number of the scales from these three tests.

6.3 **PAI:** His score on the Negative Impression scales was high. Often, this arises because the examinee is attempting to exaggerate difficulties and problems he/she has, but at the level at which JD was scoring a more likely hypothesis is that he holds an extremely negative self-construct of himself and doubts, probably on a temporary basis, his own worth. This reflects an extreme incongruity with the picture he tried to portray of himself during the interview and reflects a fundamental conflict of self-constructs which will result in conflicting motivations and attitudes.

6.4 The scale and subscales recording Somatic Complaints were significantly high due to self-report of functional impairment or symptoms associated with sensory or motor dysfunctions. There was also a more general theme to this scale indicating repeated problems, some with a relatively minor physical base, extending into nonspecific fears about health and physical functioning. This is an indication that JD, despite the tough and hardy image he seeks to portray, is actually experiencing stress at a somatic level.

6.5 The score on the Anxiety scale was high also. Scores within his range suggest significant anxiety and tension and normally the respondent is probably tense much of the time and ruminative about anticipated misfortune. Such individuals may be seen as highly-strung and dependent. In JD's case, the main effect on this scale comes from Traumatic Stress. This stress is normally the product of a disturbing or traumatic incident and produces recurrent episodes of anxiety. Respondents generally report that the event has left them changed or damaged in some fundamental way, and in this case the most likely incident causing JD such long-term difficulties is a consequence of attachment difficulties associated with his experiences of being parented. Currently, he will of course be stressed about the possible outcome of these investigations.

6.6 JD scored highly on the Mania scale which measures a tendency to elevated mood, expansiveness, heightened activity level and impatience. Specifically in his case he responded to those items that tap activity and energy level to an extent that would be noticeably high to most observers. He also responded positively to items recording a disorganised and naive manner within interpersonal behaviour.

6.7 JD also showed a high score on Antisocial Behaviours relating specifically to a history of antisocial acts manifested as conduct disorder during adolescence. Items concerning egocentricity were also responded to positively indicating that JD is constantly monitoring himself and his responses within the social world.

6.8 The results on the scales recording antisocial traits were not high enough to suggest a diagnosis of antisocial or narcissistic personality disorders, but are similar to scores associated with borderline personality disorder.

6.9 **IBS**: JD produced a high score on the General Aggressiveness Rational scale (GCR) which examines the general response class of aggressiveness over a wide variety of item content which includes aggressive behaviours, and feelings and attitudes. Many aggressive people in the workplace tend to score highly on this scale, indicating that they are prone to the use of aggression across contexts and not just in the workplace. This seems to be the case with JD who has acknowledged a history of aggression at school and in his failed marriage.

6.10 He scored highly on the Hostile Stance scale (HS) which evaluates an antagonistic approach towards other people, one where aggression is justified as a means of being successfully competitive and/or to protect oneself against possible threat.

6.11 The Verbal Aggressiveness scale (VA) is often scored highly on by aggressive managers who know how to use forcefully expressed words to create maximum psychological damage. JD scored positively on items including those relating to criticising, patronising, and putting others down.

6.12   In addition and most worryingly, he scored at a moderately high level on the Physical Aggressiveness scale (PA) which measures the tendency to use physical force in interpersonal situations or to fantasise about the use of violence. Many workplace aggressors have an elevated score on this scale because of their fantasies but never actually put themselves at risk of official action against them by physically assaulting their victims.

6.13   JD's scores on the scales of Assertiveness were either low or low average – a marked contrast to the scales recording aggressive traits and attitudes. This suggests that he uses aggression where others are more likely to use pro-social assertive behaviour. He confuses his aggression with assertion or finds it convenient to do so.

6.14   I note that JD has an extremely low score on the Praise scale. This suggests strongly that he is used to both giving and receiving little praise throughout the major settings of his life. This is again a probable reflection of dysfunctional parenting experiences and the result of modelling by distant and sometimes hostile parents who did not understand the need to show him approval through praise.

6.15   **FAST**: Suicidal Ideation was moderately elevated and congruent with his descriptions during the interview. There was no elevation on Helplessness or the behavioural dimension of suicide. This suggests that JD thinks about suicide but does not have reasons founded in a belief of helplessness to translate these thoughts into action.

7.0   *Formulation*

7.1   Harassment in the workplace is a subset of behaviours that are part of the wide range of human aggression. In common with the behaviours throughout this wide range, repeated workplace harassment has antecedents which initiate it and consequences which reinforce its continued use.

7.2   The antecedents may also be wide and varied. In most cases there are features or presumed features of the organisation which create conditions in which harassment becomes more probable. Then there may be specific difficulties within departments or sections which elicit feelings of frustration and aggression. These include insecurity about employment, stress relating to high workloads and difficult deadlines, poor staffing levels and insufficient resources.

7.3   Personal characteristics of some staff may increase the probability that they may be targeted by potential harassers. They may be comparatively good at their work, inciting jealousy, or very poor at it such that others have to support them too often. Others may be seen to be 'soft targets' because they are easily upset or passive; some may be demonstrably anxious and vulnerable.

7.4   None of these will elicit aggressive harassment from someone who is well socialised and in control of his/her emotions. Such people do not respond to frustration by becoming overtly angry even if they may feel it. In general, it is those people who are less well socialised and who have learned to respond to frustration with aggression who do so when eliciting setting conditions are present.

8.0 *Opinion*

8.1 JD's history reveals many facets which lead me to the opinion that he is poorly inhibited. His background is one of aggressive intolerance and over-control. Dysfunctional attachments characterise his formative years and appear to persist into his early adulthood; his marriage and parenting career were doomed as a consequence.

8.2 Early on, he found that aggression at school (almost certainly taking the form of bullying) resulted in positive reinforcement. His coterie of friends admired him and it is possible that he confused his bullying with a form of strong leadership. He is conflicted in terms of his own self-constructs; he portrays strength, leadership and positive management with fears about his self-worth. He has a strong sense of wanting to belong to a family or other close group but tries to hide his fears of isolation behind a façade of aggressive self-reliance.

8.3 JD's personality characteristics show markedly aggressive traits which are operative within a borderline personality disorder. Not surprisingly his interpersonal behaviour is strongly mediated by this, showing the use of aggression rather than assertion and significant disregard for the rights of others.

8.4 He is attracted to conflict – probably because his life experiences teach him that it is likely to be a winner. Being blind to his motivations he is largely unaware of the way in which others may perceive him. He still thinks of himself as a 'leader' rather than a 'bully'. He cannot reconcile these positive views with the fear of abandonment by his parents and his ex-wife.

8.5 **Borderline personality disorder**: Individuals with this disorder are generally frightened and distressed by real or imagined abandonment. Rejection by parents, spouse, partner or peers may lead to profound changes in self-constructs and produce conflicted self-perceptions. Inappropriate anger/aggression is a common trait and may be revealed in a variety of settings.

8.6 Relationships are invariably unstable and characterised by anger and aggressive outbursts. People with this disorder may switch from lauding people to devaluing them. Such support as they give seems to be part of an unstated contract that the people supported will be loyal to them no matter what the circumstances.

8.7 They show impulsivity and may have a string of driving offences, if not other more serious convictions. They often produce evidence of suicidal ideations.

8.8 People with this disorder do not cope well with perceptions of threat and other interpersonal stressors. They react angrily and are often caustic in their appraisal of those who thwart or irritate them. They can have difficulties controlling their anger and may well voice their dissatisfactions loudly.

9.0 *Recommendations*

9.1 Whether or not the allegations of the two women are substantiated; there is a clear need to review JD's management skills.

9.2 He needs therapeutic sessions, first to explore these assessment findings and secondly to help him understand the need for change. To set the scene for this work it would be helpful if a senior manager could dispel his mythical thinking that his aggressive style is valued by the organisation. (If he is right, however, and his behaviour is encouraged, then the company can expect many more complaints and litigation.)

9.3 JD needs to take part in relevant people management courses and Human Resources will be able to arrange this. He then needs a period of supervision and monitoring to ensure that he does not pay lip-service to such inputs. Review in six months is vital.

———

The second report concerns a local authority secretarial/clerical officer; one of a small team of similarly graded staff who provide services to a large technical services department. She alleged harassment by three of the six section managers whose staff required the clerical and secretarial services. She complained that they were verbally aggressive, demanding and demeaned her work. In response, they complained that she was imperious and verbally aggressive to their junior staff and constantly complaining.

Psychological Report
on
KW (Date of Birth: 11–10–66)

Clerical Officer
Technical Services
Date of Report:

1.0 *Reason for Referral*

1.1 KW was referred by the Local Authority Employee Assistance Programme. She has been on long-term sick leave with stress-related disorder, allegedly resulting from harassment within the workplace.

1.2 The alleged harassers are three section heads who are aware of the allegations. They have made counter-allegations that KW is herself harassing young junior staff in their section, refusing their work and creating unpleasant rumours.

2.0 *Summary*

2.1 This assessment was based upon information from documentation, interviews and psychometric assessments. The following recommendations were derived:

KW is a woman of normal ability who is severely debilitated by post-traumatic stress disorder and comorbid social anxiety disorder. These have arisen from a history of perceived workplace bullying and have led to significant restrictions on emotional well-being and normal functioning as wife, mother and employee.

The cognitive-behavioural programme provided by the EAP is correct and the onward psychiatric referral is desirable also as close monitoring of medication will be required.

In relation to the Judicial Studies Board Guidelines, KW's current prognosis is within the severe range and I am of the opinion that she will not be able to sustain employment within the foreseeable future.

3.0 *Basis of this assessment*

3.1 This assessment has made use of information from:

- the following documents

  (1) Referral notes, Personal
  (2) Allegations of KW
  (3) Responses to allegations summarised by Mrs CT, Human Resources
  (4) KW's job description and employment record

- five interview sessions with KW, each of one-hour duration
- psychometric testing

4.0 *Background*

4.1 **Employment record:** KW has appropriate typing, word-processing and office systems qualifications. She has been involved with office work since leaving school but had a period of eight years off to cover the early years of her three children.

4.2 KW began work with the LA two years ago. She was previously employed by an insurance broker. There are no adverse comments on her records but I note that there is no information older than three years. She has had significant sick leave since joining the LA but this has been properly documented.

4.3 KW has been on sick leave for nearly five months; she has regular sessions with an EAP counsellor and gets support from her union representative. She alleges that she has been subjected to severe verbal aggression including the use of obscenity, has had her work output criticised unfairly and repeatedly, and had been prevented from using her computer so work had passed important deadlines. She claims also that she has been discriminated against in respect of annual leave choices.

4.4 The record taken by Human Resources states that KW has suffered a nervous breakdown as a consequence of the harassment. It states that she is now unable to come back to work and is frightened of leaving her home.

4.5 Notes summarising conversations with the alleged harassers counter the allegations described above. There is a belief that it has been necessary to defend trainee staff from KW's bullying ways. There are quotes included from the two trainees who have complained about KW's attitude and demeaning remarks.

5.0 *Interview with KW*

5.1 **Circumstances of the interview:** All sessions were held in KW's home; she felt safe there and preferred that venue to the EAP offices which she claims she is too frightened to visit.

5.2 KW is a generously built woman of good average height; her demeanour is very serious and she rarely smiles. Often her posture is poor; she appears to be bent over as though under the weight of her worry.

5.3 Her presentation has been fairly 'flat', apart from outbursts of anger when discussing the harassment. These outbursts have always given way to quiet tears. KW is particularly angry that she has been 'forced' into taking medication and having therapy: 'Why should they have done this to me?'

5.4 KW was able to respond appropriately to the interview; she was fully oriented in time, place and person but showed some difficulties of episodic memory. Some dissociative thinking was evident but generally during her periods of emotional arousal.

5.5 **Personal history:** KW provided a personal history during a session structured by the Multimodal Life History Questionnaire. There were no abnormalities in her medical and developmental history but there was significant evidence of family dysfunction.

5.6 KW confirmed that she had been bullied extensively by her older sister and, after some difficulty, suggested that she had been equally harassing of her younger brother. She was finally able to state that this brother had borne the burden of the two sisters' rivalry.

5.7 She felt that this rivalry continued into school where she was bullied by her sister's friends. This carried on spasmodically for years, even after her sister had moved up to comprehensive school. KW agreed that she also got a reputation for causing trouble but claimed that this was simply her way of defending herself.

5.8 KW felt that the relationship she had with her sister was still competitive but acknowledged that they had found ways to live reasonably normally.

5.9 **Attachment history**: KW's responses to this section of the interview were analysed according to the Adult Attachment Interview. The results indicated that she experienced anxious avoidant parenting from both parents who seemed overwhelmed by the task of bringing up three children. Her responses suggested that all three children were simply bought off rather than disciplined effectively. Inconsistencies and lack of structure pervaded the parents' setting of limits. KW stated 'There was no blame and no rules.' It seemed that this style of parenting left all three children to compete unequally with each other. The youngest child seems to have borne the brunt of this, but KW showed no remorse about this, saying only 'I suppose I'm not surprised he doesn't have much to do with us [KW and her sister].'

5.10 **Employment environment:** KW described her working environment as 'hellish'. She gave a detailed description of the harassment she alleges which is identical in all significant respects to her written report. She states that there is an aggressive 'blame' culture throughout the department and believes that this comes from 'macho' leadership and a 'dog eat dog' attitude.

5.11 I asked her about her friendship pattern within the department and she named four women who she felt closer to. When asked what support they had given her, she felt that they would have, had there not been pressure put upon them.

5.12 She stated again that the prevailing culture of the department was one of repression and 'dog eat dog'. She claimed that the only way she could survive was by 'asserting herself' whenever she felt it was necessary. Eventually this strategy had failed her; she was not equal to the pressure that was exerted on her; she claimed that she was told to complete tasks with impossible deadlines and that 'I became the sacrificial lamb when it all went pear-shaped.'

5.13 She claimed that two managers and some of her own grades were the principal perpetrators. She accused the managers of being highly and unnecessarily critical; she stated that on three occasions they had prevented her from using her terminal such that work fell behind schedule and got her into trouble with other managers. The line manager responsible claims that her machine was taken out of service in a sequence pending modifications to the network. KW does not accept this explanation.

5.14 KW also alleges that she has been threatened with violence and sworn at obscenely and repeatedly. She was unwilling to name people who had done this for fear of 'further reprisals' and stated that 'they got a big kick out of it – I heard them laughing and giving each other those American high hand slaps'.

5.15   Over a period of ten months KW felt that the behaviour escalated. She became very fearful and unable to concentrate. This made her work-rate slower and earned her further criticisms. The worse she got, the more harassment she attracted. Eventually she became so stressed that she went to her GP and was diagnosed with depression and anxiety. She was given medication, including soporifics as she was having serious problems with her sleep routine.

5.16   She claims that the bullying became so severe that it generalised from the overall group of perpetrators listed above to a much broader group who would make fun of her and refer to her body weight in a humorous but hurtful way. She became embarrassed by her size, particularly when a loud conversation was designed for her to overhear in the canteen. This happened on several occasions and with similar content. Essentially, the group conversing (names supplied by KW) made points to the effect that overweight people perspired heavily and smelt; their smell and appearance were offensive and they should know better.

5.17   KW took this to heart; she showered twice a day and wore baggy clothes. She spent so much time getting ready for work that she was often late. This earned her even more criticism and anger that other people were having to pick up her work.

5.18   Her absences from the department became more frequent and eventually she was required to attend a disciplinary meeting with her line manager, section head and union representative. She stated that no one would believe her ('Probably I was overweight, not like them') and they would dismiss her abruptly when she could not collaborate her assertions or find an independent witness: 'Who would stand up for me when everyone is so scared?'

5.19   Given a lot of support she was able to attend the meeting but had to leave this meeting because she began to flush, palpitate and feel faint. She then had two days off, went back on the third day but stayed only two hours. She felt intimidated by the hostility of her line manager.

5.20   Since then, her attendance has been spasmodic and eventually failed altogether. Flashbacks, avoidance and intrusive thoughts became very familiar, gradually preventing her from effectively following through her daily functioning.

5.21   Eventually, she was placed on the special service programme of the EAP (additional support) because she was experiencing suicidal ideation. She cannot now leave her home and her husband has to do all the shopping and any domestic tasks that involve meeting other people. She experiences involuntary spasms of the arms and upper body which she calls 'shaking fits' when she leaves her home and worries that people are going to be critical of her.

5.22   KW cannot ride in their car for more than ten minutes and is finding it difficult even to visit her mother and sister; she can experience ten or more of the 'shaking fits' within a single two-hour-long visit. Activities her children are involved in have had to be cancelled unless their father is available to take them. This is often difficult because of the nature of his work.

5.23 KW describes herself as increasingly isolated and unable to communicate without stress.

5.25 **Clinician-Administered PTSD Scale for DSM-IV (CAPS)**: The CAPS questionnaire forms part of the clinical interview which is highly structured. It is designed to assess the seventeen symptoms of PTSD outlined in DSM-IV (see Formulation section below). It is used to assess severity and frequency of each symptom and so provides a comprehensive assessment of PTSD symptomatology. Its primary purpose is to enable a diagnosis of PTSD and it does provide a means to evaluate the symptoms on an individual's social and occupational functioning. The CAPS scales record symptoms of intrusion (the tendency of post-traumatic stress effects to intrude on day-to-day activities), symptoms of avoidance (the tendency of PTSD sufferers to avoid trauma associated with people and situations), symptoms of increased physiological arousal, duration of PTSD effects, and evidence of clinical distress or impairment in social, occupational or other important areas of functioning. The results on the CAPS showed that KW has significant scores on these scales and the overall result indicates chronic post-traumatic stress disorder.

5.26 **Self-perceptions**: When asked to complete the 'Images' section of the Multimodal Life History Questionnaire, KW indicated that 'Being hurt', 'Not coping', 'Losing control', 'Being laughed at' and 'Failing' applied to her. When asked to complete the 'Thoughts' section, she stated that 'Intelligent', 'Loyal', 'Trustworthy', 'Full of regrets', 'Considerate', 'Hard working', and 'Concentration problems' and 'Memory problems' applied to her.

5.27 KW thought for a long time about the 'Behaviours' section from the Questionnaire and finally aligned herself with 'Overeat', 'Drink too much', 'Procrastination', 'Sleep disturbance', 'Crying' and 'Outbursts of temper'.

6.0 *Psychometric assessment*

6.1 KW was given three psychometric schedules to complete. These are the ICES Personality Inventory (ICES), the Interpersonal Behaviour Survey (IBS) and the Impact of Events Scale (IES). The first of these is a self-administered objective inventory of adult personality designed to provide information on critical clinical variables. It is a modern and powerful inventory containing four validity scales. The second schedule (IBS) is a sensitive measure of the different ways in which people respond to others in their normal community settings. Included amongst these scales are three which deal with response types associated with the conscious or unconscious distortion of interpersonal behaviour. Thus one scale deals with denial, a second with random responding and a third with impression management (Fake good). These scales are generic in that they are associated with interpersonal behaviour generally rather than in specific relation to workplace settings. The third scale is the most widely used self-report measure of specific responses to trauma. It consists of two subscales, which record separately experiences of intrusion and avoidance. The intrusion subscale measures the extent to which memories of the traumatic event continue to impinge on the individual. The avoidance subscale measures the extent to which the individual tries to exclude unpleasant memories from consciousness and deliberately tries to avoid locations and other reminders of the event.

6.2 KW was found to have significant scores on a number of the scales from these three tests.

6.3 Her profile on the ICES showed her to be anxious, suspicious, submissive and non-confrontational, introverted, well-organised and conventional. This fits well with the 'victim' profile determined by research studies.

6.4 The IBS results showed significant other trends, however, which included a very high level on the Passive Aggressiveness scale. This is associated with indirectly aggressive behaviours such as negativism, stubbornness, procrastination and complaining. Her score on the Verbal Aggressiveness scale was high, and this records the trait of using words as weapons, perhaps by denigrating other people's efforts, making fun of them and being critical.

6.5 By contrast, KW's scores on the Assertiveness scales were low; the combination is indicative of someone who fails to assert herself when that would be desirable but complains afterwards and is generally verbally aggressive about people she perceives as thwarting her or otherwise putting pressure on her.

6.6 Such traits are soon evident to co-workers and bring about negative evaluations and loss of support.

6.7 Her score on the Dependency scale was also strongly significant and indicative of a person who needs to rely on others for decision making, and who experiences feelings of powerlessness and of loss of support. Attention-seeking behaviour is also associated with this scale.

6.8 **IES**: KW completed this test appropriately and her scores for both intrusion and avoidance exceeded 1.5 sd of the test norms. This is further indication that she is subject to severe post-traumatic stress disorder.

7.0 *Formulation and opinion*

7.1 Research indicates that many people who have experienced bullying as children from siblings and/or peers may also become victims in adult life.

7.2 It is also the case that some victims may also develop bullying behaviours, in some cases to alleviate the frustration of their failure to avoid being harassed.

7.3 Research shows also that one of the common outcomes of repeated workplace harassment is a form of post-traumatic stress disorder. The internationally agreed criteria are as follows:

7.4 The internationally agreed criteria (DSM-IV, APA, 1994) for the diagnosis of post-traumatic stress disorder (PTSD) are:

A   *The person has been exposed to a traumatic event in which both the following were present:*

(1) *the person experienced, witnessed or was confronted with an event or events that involved actual or threatened death or serious injury, or a threat to the physical integrity of self or others.*

(2) *the person's response involved intense fear, helplessness, or horror.*

B   *The traumatic event is persistently re-experienced in one or more of the following ways:*

(1) *recurrent and intrusive distressing recollections of the event, including images, thoughts, or perceptions.*

(2) *recurrent distressing dreams of the event.*

(3) *acting or feeling as if the traumatic event were recurring (includes a sense of reliving the experience, illusions, hallucinations, and dissociative flashback episodes, including those that occur on awakening or when intoxicated).*

(4) *intense psychological distress at exposure to internal or external cues that symbolise or resemble an aspect of the traumatic event.*

(5) *physiological reactivity on exposure to internal or external cues that symbolise or resemble an aspect of the traumatic event.*

C   *Persistent avoidance of stimuli associated with the trauma and numbing of general responsiveness (not present before the trauma), as indicated by three or more of the following:*

(1) *efforts to avoid thoughts, feelings, or conversations associated with the trauma*

(2) *efforts to avoid activities, places, or people that arouse recollections of the trauma*

(3) *inability to recall an important aspect of the trauma*

(4) *markedly diminished interest or participation in significant activities*

(5) *feeling of detachment or estrangement from others*

(6) *restricted range of affect*

(7) *sense of a foreshortened future (e.g. does not expect to have a career, marriage, children, or a normal life span)*

D   *Persistent symptoms of arousal, as indicated by two or more of the following:*

   (1) difficulty falling asleep or staying asleep
   (2) irritability or outbursts of anger
   (3) difficulty concentrating
   (4) hypervigilance
   (5) exaggerated startle response

E   *Duration of the disturbance (symptoms in Criteria B, C, and D) is more than 1 month.*

F   *The disturbance causes clinically significant distress or impairment in social, occupational, or other important areas of functioning.*

7.5 KW's interview responses and responses to the Impact of Events schedule indicate that she fulfils Criteria A, B1, 3 and 4, C1 and 2, D1, 2 and 4. Criteria E and F are fulfilled in respect of the recorded history as well as by her interview responses.

7.6 A further confounding factor for some victims of harassment who have suffered repeated insults about their personal characteristics is social anxiety disorder (sometimes referred to as social phobia). People who experience this behave in such a way as to significantly limit the possibilities of encountering unfamiliar or potentially difficult people; this generally means that they are unable to move freely around the community for fear of encountering such people. The internationally agreed criteria (DSM-IV) for this condition are as follows:

A   *A marked and persistent fear of one or more social or performance situations in which the person is exposed to unfamiliar people or to possible scrutiny by others. The individual fears that he or she will act in a way (or show anxiety symptoms) that will be humiliating or embarrassing.*

B   *Exposure to the feared social situation almost invariably provokes anxiety, which may take the form of situationally bound or situationally predisposed panic attack.*

C   *The person recognises that the fear is excessive or unreasonable.*

D   *The feared social or performance situations are avoided or else are endured with intense anxiety or distress.*

E   *The avoidance, anxious anticipation, or distress in the feared social or performance situation(s) interferes significantly with the person's normal routine, occupational (academic) functioning, or social activities or relationships, or there is marked distress about having the phobia.*

F   *In individuals under the age of 18 years, the duration is at least 6 months.*

G   *The fear or avoidance is not due to the direct physiological effects of a substance (e.g. a drug of abuse, a medication) or a general medical condition and is not better accounted for by another mental disorder (e.g. Panic Disorder with or without Agoraphobia, Separation Anxiety Disorder, Body Dysmorphic Disorder, a Pervasive Developmental Disorder, or Schizoid Personality Disorder).*

H *If a general medical condition or another mental disorder is present, the fear in Criterion A is unrelated to it, e.g. the fear is not of Stuttering, trembling in Parkinson's disease, or of exhibiting abnormal eating behaviour in Anorexia Nervosa or Bulimia Nervosa.*

7.6   KW satisfies the criteria for this in respect of all the criteria shown above.

7.7   KW's present psychopathology is severe and very debilitating. In relation to the Judicial Studies Board Guidelines the psychological factors to take into account are as follows:

(i)   KW's ability to cope with life and work;
(ii)   the effect on her relationships with family, friends and those with whom she comes into contact;
(iii) the extent to which treatment would be successful;
(iv)   future vulnerability;
(v)   prognosis;
(vi)   whether medical help has been sought.

7.8   As is clear from the factors listed above, KW's ability to cope with life in general is now very poor. She is entirely dependent upon her husband for all domestic and personal matters outside of the home and many of those within. In addition, she is unable to work, so her roles as wife, mother and employee have all been affected.

7.9   All her relationships have suffered and that with her husband is increasingly under strain as he is unable to comprehend fully the extent of his wife's difficulties. Although kindly, he is of the 'pull yourself together' type and so unable to support her fully. In addition, her children experience their mother as a housebound, inactive, complaining and self-centred person who no longer supports their activities.

7.10   The extent to which treatment will be successful is unknowable at present. Suggestions for this are given below and it will be very long-term. I am not optimistic that KW will recover to the extent that full normal functioning will be possible in the foreseeable future.

7.11   Even if KW does recover well in terms of daily functioning she will be a very delicate person whose memories and anxieties about the bullying will be close to the surface. She will remain vulnerable as a consequence. In addition, she will be easily stressed by workload variation and her performance is likely to be erratic. This will bring her to the attention of her colleagues whose evaluations of her are thus likely to be negative. In short, history is likely to repeat itself. I am therefore pessimistic as to whether she will be able to work again even if treatment is successful.

7.12 KW has sought medical help and has also done her best to follow the suggestions of the personnel officers and her union representatives. It is unlikely, therefore, that it could be argued that she has failed to mitigate her losses to the best of her ability.

7.13 Inevitably, therefore, I must consider the prognosis to be very poor such that she falls within the 'severe' category of the Judicial Studies Board Guidelines.

8.0 *Conclusions*

8.1 KW is a woman of normal ability who is severely debilitated by post-traumatic stress disorder and comorbid social anxiety disorder. These have arisen from a history of perceived workplace bullying and have led to significant restrictions on emotional well-being and normal functioning as wife, mother and employee.

8.2 The cognitive-behavioural programme provided by the EAP is correct and the onward psychiatric referral is desirable also as close monitoring of medication will be required.

8.3 In relation to the Judicial Studies Board Guidelines, KW's current prognosis is within the severe range and I am of the opinion that she will not be able to sustain employment within the foreseeable future.

––––––––

The model of workplace bullying

Chapter 2 put forward a model of workplace bullying based upon a multi-faceted pragmatic assembly of well-researched antecedents known to be associated with this behaviour. The two case studies provided above show complex variables associated with the bullying that was reported. Although only two cases are reported here it is the writer's experience that the variables involved are commonplace within this form of human aggression and illuminate the spectrum of individual factors that are associated with its blight on employment experience.

The second chapter proposed also that workplace bullying could be conceptualised, at least for the purposes of investigation, as the product of a variety of antecedents and reinforcing consequences in much the same way as any other form of interpersonal human aggression. These included external settings such as the effects of the physical environment, the culture of the organisation, aggressive norms and job type. Setting conditions include external factors such as stressful and frustrating conditions, restructuring and redundancy, whilst internal factors include unpleasant feelings, hostile attributional bias, cognitions associated with Type A behaviour patterns and difficulties of self-monitoring. Specific events acting as antecedents include unfair treatment, unreasonable demands and various forms of victim trait behaviour. The model concludes with the specification of reinforcing events which promote and strengthen the behaviour of bullying.

The case study of JD reveals factors that can be placed within the model which implicitly guided the assessment. These can be summarised with reference to the depiction of the model in Figure 2 in Chapter 2 (see p. 52):

Settings external	JD perceived an aggressive culture which reinforced the forceful treatment of employees who were thought to be slack and poor time-keepers.
Setting conditions – external	JD described stressful conditions arising from restructuring and staff appraisal. There was an implied threat of redundancy to staff.
Setting conditions – internal	JD showed considerable bias to hostile attribution in the comments made about the complainants. In addition, he expressed a series of aggressive thoughts relating to unpleasant feelings he held about his relationship with others. His self-monitoring was poor because he was unable to assess the impact of his words on others. He had conflicting self-constructs which emanated from dysfunctional attachment, fear of abandonment/ isolation and faulty social learning going back to peer reinforcement during his school days.
Specific events:	He assumed provocation and perceived common signs of victim trait behaviour; e.g. 'Both are always moaning and complaining'; 'brought to book by two slackers'.
Bullying behaviour	A range of threatening and intimidatory behaviour, not uncommon within the behavioural spectrum of workplace bullying.
Reinforcement	Dominance, self-reinforcement of self as a strong leader, vicarious experience of reinforcement by peers (school days) and stress/frustration reduction.

This analysis identifies the factors that need to be corrected. As can be seen, this involves adjusting the workplace ethic that enables aggression to be used as a management strategy; it also involves a significant amount of therapeutic input with JD to help him come to terms with the fears that bedevil him and which he has been seeking to placate by acting as a strong leader who confuses aggression with firmness.

KW's case can be subjected to the same analysis. This seems to be less straightforward as she is both a victim and a bully; her prognosis at the level of psychopathology is poor and she is unlikely to return to work in the medium-term future.

Settings – external	She alleges a 'dog eat dog' culture with aggressive norms and repressive traits.
Setting conditions – external	Loss of peer support.
Setting conditions – Internal	Unpleasant feelings. Hostile thoughts about junior staff.
Specific events	Being harassed, made a scapegoat and having unreasonable demands placed upon her.
Behaviour	As stated above, she made allegations of severe bullying but others made similar claims against her.
Reinforcement	For her the subjugation of juniors was a form of dominance; there is no information about these factors in respect of those who bullied her but there is a strong suggestion of peer approval for them (see para. 5.14).

As described, this model of workplace bullying appears to be useful as a means of guiding an investigation of adult bullying within the workplace. It is not, however, as specific as its contents would suggest; the headings could remain constant but many of the particular exemplars could be changed to meet other environments where humans come together –the community, the home, the charity workshop, the parish council meeting. Tragically, bullying is an abuse of power that finds its way into virtually every sphere of communal human endeavour. The opening of Chapter 2 suggested that we can blind ourselves to the comforting restraints of context specificity; in so doing we are able to view workplace bullying as a unique phenomenon that is a product of adults functioning badly within the particular environs of employment. Yet the model of workplace aggression put forward within that chapter is little more than a series of boxed headings with lists of particular antecedent or reinforcing factors. It takes only a brief glance to realise that these headings are not peculiar to workplace aggression. They may be used for almost all varieties of human aggression; the lists beneath may change but the principal ingredients are the same. This is easy to overlook by limiting study purely to one context of human aggression or another.

When one considers the staggering fact that one person in the UK is assaulted every twenty seconds – a better situation than that experienced by the inhabitants of many other countries including the US – then there is a moral duty on the part of researchers to step outside narrow fields of interest for a time and consider the broader picture. There is little escape from the fact that workplace bullying is not a unitary phenomenon; it is merely a part of that broader picture. The only variation is within the nature of external settings and setting conditions; the lists under the headings, the internal setting conditions and the motivations are hardly different; bullying remains an abuse of power and an intention to cause harm through the deliberate use of aggression no matter where it is found.

References

Adams, A. (1992) *Bullying at Work*, London: Virago.

Ainsworthy, M.D.S., Blehar, M.C., Waters, E. and Wall, S. (1978) *Patterns of Attachment: A Psychological Study of the Strange Situation*, Hillsdale, NJ: Lawrence Erlbaum.

Allen, J.G. (1981) The clinical psychologist as a diagnostic consultant, *Bulletin of the Menninger Clinic*, 45, 247–258.

Allgulander, C. (1999) Paroxetine in social anxiety disorder: a randomised placebo-controlled study, *Acta Psychiatrica Scandinavia*, 100, 193–198.

Aluja-Fabregat, A. and Torrubia-Beltri, R. (1998) Viewing of mass media violence, perception of violence, personality and academic achievement, *Personality and Individual Differences*, 25, 973–989.

Amaya-Jackson, L. and March, J.S. (1995) Posttraumatic stress disorder. In J.S. March (ed.) *Anxiety Disorders in Children and Adolescents*, New York: Guilford Press, pp. 276–300.

Ambert, J.G. (1994) *Coping with Trauma: A Guide to Self-understanding*, Washington, DC: American Psychiatric Press.

American Psychiatric Association (1994) *Diagnostic and Statistical Manual of Mental Disorders* (4th edition) (DSM–IV), Washington, DC: American Psychiatric Association.

Anderson, C.A., Anderson, K.B. and Deuser, W.E. (1996) Violent crime rate studies in philosophical context: a destructive testing approach to heat and southern culture of violence effects, *Personality and Social Psychology Bulletin*, 22, 366–376.

Anderson, C.A., Deuser, W.E. and DeNeve, K.M. (1995) Hot temperatures, hostile affect, hostile cognition, and arousal: tests of a general model of affective aggression, *Personality and Social Psychology Bulletin*, 21, 434–448.

Appelberg, K., Romanov, V., Honlasalo, M. and Koskenvuo, M. (1991) Interpersonal conflicts at work and psychosocial characteristics of employees, *Social Science Medicine*, 32, 1051–1056.

Augustinous, M. and Walker, I. (1995) *Social Cognition: An Integrated Introduction*, London: Sage.

Austin, S. and Joseph, S. (1996) Assessment of bully–victim problems in 8 to 11 year-olds, *British Journal of Educational Psychology*, 66, 447–456.

Baldry, A.C. and Farrington, D.P. (2000) Bullies and delinquents: personal characteristics and parental styles, *Journal of Community and Applied Social Psychology*, 10, 17–31.

Bandura, A. (1977) *Social Learning Theory*, Englewood Cliffs, New Jersey: Prentice Hall.

Bandura, A. (1978) Learning and behavioral theories of aggression. In I.L. Kutash, S.B. Kutash and L.B. Schlesinger *et al.* (eds) *Violence: Perspectives on Murder and Aggression*, New York: Academic Press.

Bandura, A. (1983) Psychological mechanisms in aggression. In R.G. Geen and E.I. Donnerstein (eds) *Aggression: Theoretical and Empirical Issues*, New York: Academic Press.

Bandura, A., Ross, D. and Ross, A. (1961) Transmission of aggression through imitation of aggressive models, *Journal of Abnormal Social Psychology*, 63, 575–582.

Baron, R.A. (1997) *Human Aggression*, New York: Plenum.

Baron, R.A. and Neuman, J.H. (1996) Workplace violence and workplace aggression: evidence on their relative frequency and potential causes, *Aggressive Behavior*, 22, 161–173.

Baron, R.A., Neuman, J.H. and Geddes, D. (1999) Evidence for the impact of perceived injustice and the Type A behavior pattern, *Aggressive Behavior*, 25, 281–296.

Baron-Cohen, S. (1989) The autistic child's theory of mind: a case of specific developmental delay, *Journal of Child Psychology and Psychiatry*, 30, 285–297.

Bartram, D. (1993) Validation of the 'ICES' personality inventory, *European Review of Applied Psychology*, 43, 207–218.

Bartram, D. (1994) *PREVUE Assessment Technical Manual* (3rd edn), Vancouver, BC: Prevue Assessments International.

Bassman, E. (1992) *Abuse in the Workplace*, Westport, CT: Quorum Books.

Baumrind, D. (1967) Child care practices anteceding three patterns of preschool behaviour, *Genetic Psychology Monographs*, 75, 43–88.

Beck, A.T., Ward, C.H., Mendelson, M., Mock, J. and Erbaugh, J. (1961) An inventory for measuring depression, *Archives of General Psychiatry*, 4, 561–571.

Bell, P.A. (1981) Physiological comfort, performance and social effects of heat-stress, *Journal of Social Issues*, 37, 71–94.

Benjamin, L.T. (1985) Defining aggression. An exercise for classroom discussion, *Teaching of Psychology*, 12, 40–42.

Ben-Porath, Y.S. (1997) Use of personality assessment instruments in empirically guided treatment planning, *Psychological Assessment*, 9, 361–367.

Berkowitz, L. (1983) The experience of anger as a parallel process in the display of impulsive 'angry' aggression. In R.G. Green and E. Donnerstein (eds) *Aggression— Theoretical and Empirical Reviews, Volume 1 – Theoretical and Methodological Issues*, New York: Academy Press, pp. 103–133.

Berkowitz, L. (1989) Frustration-aggression hypothesis: examination and reformulation, *Psychological Bulletin*, 106, 59–73.

Billings, A.G. and Moos, R.H. (1985) Children of parents with unipolar depression: a controlled 1 year follow-up, *Journal of Abnormal Child Psychology*, 14, 149–166.

Bjorkqvist, K., Osterman, K. and Hjelt-Bäck, M. (1994) Aggression among university employees, *Aggressive Behavior*, 20, 173–184.

Bjorkqvist, K., Osterman, K. and Kaukiainen, A. (2000) Social intelligence minus empathy = aggression, *Aggression and Violent Behavior*, 5, 191–200.

Bjorkqvist, K., Osterman, K. and Largerspetz, K.M.J. (1994) Sex differences in covert aggression among adults, *Aggressive Behavior*, 20, 27–33.

Blanchard, D.C., Herbert, M., Blanchard, R.J. (1999) Continuity versus correctness: animal models and human aggression. In M. Haug and R.E. Whalen (eds) *Animal Models of Human Emotion and Cognition*, Washington, DC: American Psychological Association.

Block, J.H., Block, J. and Morrison, A. (1981) Parental agreement–disagreement on child-personality correlates in children, *Child Development*, 52, 965–974.

Booth, C.L., Rose-Krasnor, L., McKinnon, J.A. and Rubin, K.H. (1994) Predicting social adjustment in middle childhood: the role of preschool attachment security and maternal style, *Social Development*, 3, 189–204.

Booth, C.L., Rose-Krasnor, L. and Rubin, K.H. (1991) Relating preschoolers' social competence and their mothers' parenting behaviours to early attachment security and high-risk status, *Journal of Social and Personal Relationships*, 8, 363–382.

Borden, R.J. (1975) Witnessed aggression: influence of an observer's sex and values on aggressive values on responding, *Journal of Personality and Social Psychology*, 31, 567–573.

Bowers, L., Smith, P.K. and Binney, V. (1994) Perceived family relationships of bullies, victims, and bully/victims in middle childhood, *Journal of Social and Personal Relationships*, 11, 215–232.

Bowlby, J. (1973) *Attachment and Loss: Separation, Anxiety and Anger*, New York: Basic Books.

Branwhite, T. (1994) Bullying and student distress: beneath the tip of the iceberg, *Educational Psychology*, 14, 59–71.

Brennan, P., Mednick, S. and Kandel, E. (1991) Congenital determinants of violent and property offending. In D.J. Pepler and K.H. Rubin (eds) *The Development and Treatment of Childhood Aggression*, Hillsdale, NJ: Lawrence Erlbaum.

Bretherton, I., Fritz, J., Zahn-Waxler, C. and Ridgeway, D. (1986) Learning to talk about emotion: a functionalist perspective, *Child Development*, 57, 529–548.

Brodsky, C.M. (1976) *The Harassed Worker*, Toronto: Lexington Books, DC Heath and Co.

Burke, J., Borus, J., Burns, B., Millstein, K. and Beaslet, M. (1982) Changes in children's behaviour after a natural disaster, *American Journal of Psychiatry*, 139, 1010–1014.

Burns, P. (1986) *Child Development*, London: Croom Helm.

Buss, A.H. (1961) *The Psychology of Aggression*, New York: Wiley.

Byrne, B.J. (1994) Bullies and victims in the school setting with reference to some Dublin schools, *The Irish Journal of Psychology*, 15, 173–184.

Cairns, R.B., Laung, M.C., Buchannan, L. and Cairns, B.D. (1995) Friendships and social networks in childhood and adolescence: fluidity, reliability, and inter-relations, *Child Development*, 66, 1330–1345.

Campbell, S. (1990) *Behavioural Problems in Preschool Children: Clinical and Developmental Issues*, New York: Guilford Press.

Campos, J., Barrett, K., Lamb, M., Goldsmith, H. and Steinberg, C. (1983) Socio-emotional development. In P.H. Mussen (ed.) *Handbook of Child Psychology* (Vol. 11), New York: Wiley, pp. 793–916.

Castle, D.J. and Morkell, D. (2000) Imagined ugliness: a symptom which can become a disorder, *Medical Journal of Australia*, 173, 205–207.

Catalano, R., Novaco, R. and McConnell, W. (1997) A model of the net effect of job loss on violence, *Journal of Personality and Social Psychology*, 72, 1440–1447.

Cicchetti, D., Cummings, E.M., Greenberg, M. and Marvin, R. (1990) An organizational perspective on attachment beyond infancy: implications for theory, measurement and research. In M. Cummings (ed.) *Attachment in the Preschool Years*, Chicago: University of Chicago Press.

Cicchetti, D., Ganiban, J. and Barnett, D. (1990) Contributions from the study of high risk populations to understanding the development of emotion regulation. In K. Dodge and J. Garber (eds) *The Development of Emotion Regulation*, New York: Cambridge University Press.

Cohn, D.A. (1990) Child–mother attachment of six-year-olds and social competence at school, *Child Development*, 61, 152–162.

Cohn, E.G. and Rotton, J. (1997) Assault as a function of time and temperature: a moderator-variable time-series analysis, *Journal of Personality and Social Psychology*, 72, 1322–1334.

Cone, J.D. (1978) The Behavioral Assessment Grid (BAG): a conceptual framework and a taxonomy, *Behavior Therapy*, 9, 882–888.

Conger, R.D., Conger, K.J., Elder, G.H., Lorenz, F., Simons, R. and Whitbeck, L. (1992) A family process model of economic hardship and adjustment of early adolescent boys, *Child Development*, 63, 526–541.

Cox, M. and Theilgaard, A. (1987) *Mutative Metaphors in Psychotherapy: The Aeolian Mode*, London: Tavistock.

Cox, M.J., Owen, M., Lewis, J.M. and Henderson, V.K. (1989) Marriage, adult adjustment and parenting, *Child Development*, 60, 1015–1024.

Cox, T. and Leather, P.J. (1994) The prevention of violence at work, *International Review of Industrial and Organizational Psychology*, 9, 213–245.

Coyne, I., Seigne, E. and Randall, P.E. (2000a) Personality traits as a predictor of workplace bully-victim status, *Proceedings of the British Psychological Society Occupational Psychology Conference*, pp. 193–198.

Coyne, I., Seigne, E. and Randall, P.E. (2000b) Predicting workplace victim status from personality, *European Journal of Work and Organizational Psychology*, 9, 335–349.

Crawford, N. (1992) The psychology of the bully. In A. Adams, *Bullying at Work*, London: Virago.

Crossley, M.L. (2000) Narrative psychology, trauma and the study of self/identity, *Theory and Psychology*, 10, 527–546.

Cummings, M. (1990) *Attachment in the Preschool Years*, Chicago: University of Chicago Press.

Davidson, J. and Smith, R. (1990) Traumatic experiences in psychiatric outpatients, *Journal of Traumatic Stress*, 3, 459–474.

Davidson, L.M. and Baum, A. (1990) Posttraumatic stress in children following natural and man-made trauma. In M.Lewis and S. Miller (eds) *Handbook of Developmental Psychopathology*, New York: Plenum, pp. 251–260.

Department for Education and Employment (1994) Circular 8/94 'Pupil Behaviour and Discipline', London: HMSO.

Dodge, K.A. and Coie, J.D. (1987) Social-information-processing factors in reactive and proactive aggression in children's peer groups, *Journal of Personality and Social Psychology*, 53, 1146–1158.

Dodge, K.A. and Frame, C.L. (1982) Social cognitive biases and deficits in aggressive boys, *Child Development*, 53, 620–635.

Dodge, K.A., Price, J.M., Bachorowski, J.A. and Newman, J.P. (1990) Hostile attributional biases in severely aggressive adolescents, *Journal of Abnormal Psychology*, 99, 385–392.

Dodge, K.A., Price, J.M., Coie, J.D. and Christopoulus, C. (1990) On the development of aggressive dyadic relationships in boys' peer groups, *Human Development*, 33, 260–270.

Dollard, J., Doob, L., Miller, N., Mowrer, O.H. and Sears, R.R. (1939) *Frustration and Aggression*, New Haven, CT: Yale University Press.

Dooley, D. and Catalano, J.C. (1988) Recent research on the psychological effects of unemployment, *Journal of Social Issues*, 44, 1–12.

Downey, G. and Coyne, J.C. (1990) Children of depressed parents: an integrative review, *Psychological Bulletin*, 108, 50–76.

Dryer, D.C. and Horowitz, L.M. (1997) When do opposites attract? Interpersonal complementarity versus similarity, *Journal of Personality and Social Psychology*, 72, 592–603.

Duncan, R.D. (1999) Peer and sibling aggression: an investigation of intra- and extra-familial bullying, *Journal of Interpersonal Violence*, 14, 871–886.

Dunn, J. (1992) Siblings and development, *Current Directions in Psychological Science*, 1(1), 6–9.

Edelmann, R.J. and Woodall, L. (1997) Bullying at work, *Occupational Psychologist*, 32, 28–31.

Edgecumbe, R. and Sandler, J. (1974) Some comments on 'Aggression turned against the self', *International Journal of Psychoanalysis*, 55, 365–368.

Einarsen, S. (1999) The nature and causes of bullying at work, *International Journal of Manpower*, 20, 16–27.

Einarsen, S. (2000) Harassment and bullying at work: a review of the Scandinavian approach, *Aggression and Violent Behavior*, 5, 379–401.

Einarsen, S. and Raknes, B.I. (1997) Harassment at work and the victimization of men, *Violence and Victims*, 12, 247–263.

Einarsen, S., Raknes, B.I. and Matthiesen, S.B. (1994) Bullying and harassment at work and its relationship with work environment quality: an exploratory study, *European Work and Organizational Psychologist*, 4, 381–401.

Einarsen, S. and Skogstad, A. (1996) Bullying at work: epidemiological findings in public and private organisations, *European Journal of Work and Organizational Psychology*, 5, 185–201.

Eisenberg, N. and Mussen, P. (1989) *The Roots of Prosocial Behaviour in Children*, Cambridge: Cambridge University Press.

Ekman, P. and Oster, H. (1979) Facial expressions of emotion, *Annual Review of Psychology*, 30, 527–554.

Elbedour, S., Ten Besel, R. and Maniyarna, G.M. (1993) Children at risk: psychological coping with war and conflict in the Middle East, *International Journal of Mental Health*, 22, 33–52.

Elton Report (1989) *Discipline in Schools*, DES and Welsh Office: HMSO.

Emde, R. (1985) The prerepresentational self and its affective core, *Psychoanalytic Study of the Child*, 38, 165–192.

Erickson, M.F., Sroufe, L.A. and Egeland, B. (1985) The relationship between quality of attachment and behaviour problems in preschool in a high-risk sample. In I. Bretherton and E. Waters (eds) Growing points in attachment theory and research, *Monographs of the Society for Research in Child Development*, 50, 147–166.

Eron, L.D., Huesmann, L.R., Dubow, E., Romanoff, R. and Yarmel, P.W. (1987) Aggression and its correlates over 22 years. In D.H. Gowell, I.M. Evans and C.R. O'Donnell (eds) *Childhood Aggression and Violence*, New York: Plenum.

Eth, S. and Pynoos, R.S. (eds) (1985) *Post Traumatic Stress Disorder in Children*, Los Angeles, CA: American Psychiatric Association.

Fagot, B. and Hagan, R. (1985) Aggression in toddlers: response to the assertive acts of boys and girls, *Sex Roles*, 12, 341–351.

Famularo, R., Fenton, T. and Kinscherff, R. (1993) Child maltreatment and the development of posttraumatic stress disorder, *American Journal of Diseases of Children*, 147, 755–760.

Felson, R.B. (1992) 'Kick'em when they're down': explanations of the relationships between stress and interpersonal aggression and violence, *Sociological Quarterly*, 33, 1–16.

Felson, R.B. and Tedeschi, J.T. (1993) *Aggression and Violence: Social Interactionist Perspectives*, Washington, DC: American Psychological Association.

Ferguson, T.J. and Rule, B.G. (1983) An attributional perspective on anger and aggression. In R.G. Green and E. Donnerstein (eds) *Aggression – Theoretical and Empirical Reviews, Volume 1 – Theoretical and Methodological Issues*, New York: Academic Press, pp. 41–74.

Feshbach, S. (1964) The function of aggression and the regulation of aggressive drive, *Psychological Review*, 71, 257–272.

Field, T. (1997) *Bully in Sight*, Wantage: Success Unlimited.

Finn, S.E. and Tonsager, M.E. (1997) Information-gathering and therapeutic models of assessment: complementary paradigms, *Psychological Assessment*, 9, 374–385.

Finnegan, R.A., Hodges, E.V.E. and Perry, D.G. (1997) Victimisation in the peer group: associations with children's perceptions of mother–child interaction, paper presented at SRCD Conference, Washington, DC.

Fischer, C.T. (1994) *Individualizing Psychological Assessment*, Hillsdale, NJ: Lawrence Erlbaum.

Fitzpatrick, G. (1995) Assessing treatability. In P. Reder and C. Lucey, *Assessment in Parenting: Psychiatric and Psychological Contributions*, London: Routledge.

Frank, A.W. (1993) The rhetoric of self-change: illness experience as narrative, *Sociological Quarterly*, 34, 39–52.

Frederick, C.J. (1985) Selected foci in the spectrum of posttraumatic stress disorders. In J. Laube and S.A. Murphy (eds) *Perspectives on Disaster Recovery*, East Norwalk: Appleton Century Crofts, pp. 110–130.

Freud, A. (1968) *Normality and Pathology in Childhood*, Harmondsworth: Penguin.

Frude, N. (1992) *Understanding Family Problems*, Chichester: Wiley.

Gable, S. and Shindledecker, R. (1993) Parental substance abuse and its relationship to severe aggression and antisocial behaviour in youth, *American Journal of Addictions*, 2(1), 40–58.

Gandolfo, R. (1995) MMPI-2 profiles of workers' compensation complainants who present with complaints of harassment, *Journal of Clinical Psychology*, 51, 711–715.

Gardner, F.E. (1989) Inconsistent parenting: is there evidence for a link with children's conduct problems, *Journal of Abnormal Child Psychology*, 17, 223–233.

Geen, R.G. (1990) *Human Aggression*, Milton Keynes: Open University Press.

Gelfand, D.M. and Teti, D.E. (1990) The effects of maternal depression on children, *Clinical Psychological Review*, 10, 329–353.

Gerard, A.B. (1994) *Parent–Child Relationship Inventory (PCRI)*, California: WPS.

Gibb, C. and Randall, P.E. (1989) *Professionals and Parents: Managing Children's Behaviour*, London: Macmillan.

Goldberg, D. and Williams, P. (1988) *A User's Guide to the General Health Questionnaire*, Windsor: NFER-Nelson.

Gould, M.S., Fisher, P., Parides, M., Flory, M. and Shaffer, D. (1996) Psychosocial risk factors of child and adolescent completed suicide, *Archives of General Psychiatry*, 53, 1155–1162.

Govia, J.M and Velicer, W.F. (1985) Comparison of multidimensional measures of aggression, *Psychological Reports*, 57, 207–215.

Green, A. (1983) Dimensions of psychological trauma in abused children, *Journal of the American Academy of Child and Adolescent Psychiatry*, 22, 231–237.

Greenberg, M.T. and Speltz, M.C. (1988) Contributions of attachment theory to the understanding of conduct problems during the preschool years. In J. Belsky and T. Nezworski (eds) *Clinical Implications of Attachment*, Hillsdale, NJ: Lawrence Erlbaum.

Harding, C. (1983) Acting with intention: a framework for examining the development of the intention to communicate. In L. Feagans, C. Garvey and R. Golinkoff (eds) *The Origins and Growth of Communication*, Norwood, NJ: Ablex.

Hargreaves, D.H. (1980) A sociological critique of individualism in education, *British Journal of Educational Studies*, 28, 187–198.

Harkness, A. R. and Lilienfeld, S.O. (1997) Individual differences sciences for treatment planning: personality traits, *Psychological Assessment*, 9, 349–360.

Hauerwas, S. (1993) *Naming the Silences: God, Medicine and the Problem of Suffering*, Edinburgh: T and T Clark.

Hawker, D.S.I. and Boulton, M.J. (2000) Twenty years of research on peer victimization and psychosocial maladjustment: a meta-analytic review of cross-sectional studies, *Journal of Child Psychology and Psychiatry*, 41, 441–455.

Heimberg, R.G., Hope, D.A., Dodge, C.S. *et al.* (1990) DSM–III–R subtypes of social phobia: comparison of generalized social phobics and public speaking phobics, *Journal of Nervous and Mental Disease*, 178, 172–179.

Herbert, M. (1985) *Caring For Your Children: A Practical Guide*, London: Blackwell.

Hinde, R.A., Tamplin, A. and Barret, J. (1993) Social-isolation in 4-year-olds, *British Journal of Developmental Psychology*, 11, 211–236.

Hodges, E.V.E. and Perry, D.G. (1999) Personal and interpersonal antecedents and consequences of victimization by peers, *Journal of Personality and Social Psychology*, 76, 677–685.

Hoel, H., Rayner, C. and Cooper, C.L. (1999) Workplace bullying, *International Review of Industrial and Organizational Psychology*, 14, 189–230.

Horowitz, M.J., Wilner, N. and Alvarez, M.A. (1979) Impact of Event Scale: a measure of subjective distress, *Psychosomatic Medicine*, 41, 207–218.

Hull, C.L. (1934) The concept of the habit-forming hierarchy and maze learning, *Psychological Review*, 41, 33–54.

Hymel, S., Woody, A. and Bowker, A. (1993) Social withdrawal in childhood: Considering the child's perspective. In K.H. Rubin and J.B. Asendropf (eds) *Social*

Withdrawal, Inhibition and Shyness in Childhood, Hillsdale, NJ: Lawrence Erlbaum, pp. 237–262.

Jaffe, L. (1988) The selected response procedure: a variation on Appelbaum's altered atmosphere procedure for the Rorschach, *Journal of Personality Assessment*, 52, 530–538.

Jenkins, C.D. (1975) The coronary-prone personality. In W.D. Gentry and R.B. Williams, Jnr. (eds) *Psychological Aspects of Myocardial and Coronary Care*, St Louis: Mosby.

Jenkins, C.D., Zyzanski, S.J. and Rosenman, R.H. (1979) *Jenkins Activity Survey Manual*, San Antonio, CA: The Psychological Corporation.

Jolanta, J.R.J. and Tomasz, M.S. (2000) The links between body dysmorphic disorder and eating disorders, *European Psychiatry*, 15, 302–305.

Jones, J.C. and Barlow, D.H. (1990) The etiology of post traumatic stress disorder, *Clinical Psychology Review*, 10, 299–328.

Jouriles, E.N., Murphy, C.M., Farris, A.M., Smith, D.A., Richters, J.E. and Waters, E. (1991) Marital adjustment, parental disagreements about child rearing and behaviour problems in boys: increasing the specificity of the marital assessment, *Child Development*, 62, 1424–1433.

Judicial Studies Board (2000) *Guidelines for the Assessment of General Damages in Personal Injury* (5th edn), London: Blackstone Press.

Kagan, J. (1974) Developmental and methodological considerations in the study of aggression. In J. deWit and W.W. Hartup (eds) *Determinants and Origins of Aggressive Behaviour*, The Hague: Mouton.

Kaukiainen, A., Bjorkqvist, K., Largerspetz, K., Osterman, K., Salmivalli, C., Rothberg, S. and Ahlbom, A. (1999) The relationships between social intelligence, empathy, and three types of aggression, *Aggressive Behavior*, 25, 81–89.

Keashly, L. (1998) Emotional abuse in the workplace, *Journal of Emotional Abuse*, 1, 85–117.

Kessler, R.C., McGonagle, K., Zhao, S. *et al.* (1994) Lifetime and 12-months prevalence of DSM-III-R psychiatric disorders in the United States: results from the National Comorbidity Survey, *Archives of General Psychiatry*, 51, 8–19.

Kessler, R.C., Stein, M.B. and Berglund, P. (1998) Social phobia subtypes in the National Comorbidity Survey, *American Journal of Psychiatry*, 155, 613–619.

Klinnert, M., Campos, J.J., Sorce, J., Emde, R. and Svejda, M. (1983) Emotions as behaviour regulators: social referencing in infancy. In R. Plutchik and H. Kellerman (eds) *Emotions in Early Development: Vol. 2: The Emotions*, New York: Academic Press.

Kochanska, G. (1993) Towards a synthesis of parental socialization and child temperament in early development of conscience, *Child Development*, 64, 325–347.

Konovsky, M.A. and Brockner, J. (1993) Managing victim and survivor layoff reactions: a procedural justice perspective. In R. Cropanzano (ed.) *Justice in the Workplace*, Hillsdale, NJ: Lawrence Erlbaum, pp. 133–153.

Kopp, C. (1982) The antecedents of self-regulation, *Developmental Psychology*, 18, 199–214.

Kumpulainen, K., Rasanen, E. and Henttonen, I. (1999) Children involved in bullying: psychological disturbance and the persistence of the involvement, *Child Abuse and Neglect*, 23, 1253–1262.

Ladd, G.W. and Ladd, B.K. (1994) Parenting behaviors and parent–child relationships: correlates of peer victimization in kindergarten? *Developmental Psychology*, 34, 1450–1458.

Lamborn, S.D., Mounts, M.S., Steinberg, L. and Dornbusch, S.M. (1991) Patterns of competence and adjustment among adolescents from authoritative, authoritarian, indulgent and neglectful families, *Child Development*, 62, 1049–1065.

Landy, S. and Peters, R. DeV. (1992) Aggressive behaviour during the preschool years. In R. DeV. Peters, R.L. McMahon, V.L. Quinsey (eds) *Aggression and Violence Throughout the Life Span*, Newbury Park, CA: Sage.

Lawler, E.J. and Thye, S.R. (1999) Bringing emotions into social exchange theory, *Annual Review of Sociology*, 25, 217–244.

Lazarus, A.A. (1973) On assertive behavior: a brief note, *Behavior Therapy*, 4, 697–699.

Lazarus, A. and Lazarus, C.N. (1991) *Multimodal Life History Questionnaire*, DeKalb, IL: Psytec Inc.

Leather, P. and Lawrence, C. (1995) Perceiving pub violence: the symbolic influence of social and environmental factors, *British Journal of Social Psychology*, 34, 395–407.

Leighton, P. (1999) Violence at work: the legal framework. In P. Leather, C. Brady, C. Lawrence, D. Beale and T. Cox (eds) *Work-Related Violence*, London: Routledge.

LeMare, L. and Rubin, K.H. (1987) Perspective taking and peer interactions: structural and developmental analyses, *Child Development*, 58, 306–315.

Lempers, J.D., Clark-Lempers, D. and Simons, R.L. (1989) Economic hardship, parenting and distress in adolescence, *Child Development*, 60, 25–39.

Lépine, J.P. and Pélissolo, A. (2000) Why take social anxiety disorder seriously, *Depression and Anxiety*, 11, 87–92.

Leymann, H. (1992) *From Mobbing to Expulsion in Working Life*, Stockholm: Publica.

Leymann, H. (1996) Mobbing and psychological terror at workplaces, *European Journal of Work and Organizational Psychology*, 5, 119–126.

Leymann, H. and Gustafsson, A. (1996) Mobbing at work and the development of post-traumatic stress disorders, *European Journal of Work and Organizational Psychology*, 5, 251–275.

Liefooghe, A.P.D. and Olafsson, R. (1999) 'Scientists' and 'amateurs': mapping the bullying domain, *International Journal of Manpower*, 20, 39–49.

Linares, L.O., Groves, B.M., Greenberg, J., Bronfman, E., Augustyn, M. and Zuckerman, B. (1999) Restraining orders: a frequent marker of adverse maternal health, *Paediatrics*, 104, 249–257.

Lipovsky, J.A. (1991) Post-traumatic stress disorder in children, *Family Community Health*, 14, 42–51.

Lipsitt, L. (1990) Fetal development in the drug age, *Child Behaviour and Development Letter*, 6, 1–3.

Lipsitt, P.D., Buka, S. and Lipsitt, L. (1990) Early intelligence scores and subsequent delinquency, *American Journal of Family Therapy*, 18, 197–208.

Lockhart, K. (1997) Experience from a staff support service, *Journal of Community and Applied Social Psychology*, 7, 193–198.

Lorenz, K. (1966) *On Aggression*, New York: Harcourt, Brace and World.

Lyons-Ruth, K., Alpern, L. and Repacholi, B. (1993) Disorganised infant attachment classification and maternal psychosocial problems as predictors of hostile-aggressive behaviour in the preschool classroom, *Child Development*, 64, 572–585.

Lytton, J. (1990) Child and parent effects in boys' behaviour disorder: a reinterpretation, *Developmental Psychology*, 26, 683–697.

MacDonald, K. and Parke, R.D. (1984) Bridging the gap: parent–child play interaction and peer interactive competence, *Child Development*, 55, 1265–1277.

McGulliciddy-deLisi, A.V. (1982) Parental beliefs about developmental processes, *Human Development*, 2, 5, 192–200.

Mackinnonlewis, C., Lamb, M.E., Arbuckle, B., Baradaran, L.P. and Volling, B.L. (1992) The relationship between biased maternal and filial attributions and the aggressiveness of their interactions, *Development and Psychopathology*, 4, 403–415.

McNally, R.J. (1991) Assessment of post-traumatic stress disorder in children, *Psychological Assessment*, 3, 531–537.

McQuire, J. and Richman, N. (1986) The prevalence of behaviour problems in three types of pre-school groups, *Journal of Child Psychology and Psychiatry*, 27, 455–472.

Mahler, M., Pine, F. and Bergman, A. (1975) *The Psychological Birth of the Human Infant*, New York: Basic Books.

Main, M., Kaplan, M. and Cassidy, J. (1985) Security in infancy, childhood and adulthood: a move to the level of representation. In I. Bretherton and E. Waters (eds) Growing points of attachment theory and research, *Monographs of the Society for Research in Child Development*, 50 (1–2, Serial no. 209), 66–102.

Marcus, R., Roke, E. and Bruner, C. (1985) Verbal and non-verbal empathy and prediction of social behaviour of young children, *Perceptual and Motor Skills*, 60, 299–309.

Martin, B. (1975) Parent–child relations. In F. Horowitz (ed.) *Review of Child Development Research*, Chicago: University of Chicago Press.

Matarazzo, J.D. (1983) The reliability of psychiatric and psychological diagnosis, *Clinical Psychology Review*, 3, 103–145.

Matas, L., Arend, R.A. and Sroufe, L.A. (1978) Continuity of adaptation in the second year: the relationship between quality of such attachment and later competence, *Child Development*, 67, 1305–1317.

Mauger, P.A. and Adkinson, D.R. (1980) *Interpersonal Behavior Survey (IBS)*, Los Angeles: WPS.

Mehta, J.K. (2000) Bullying in the workplace: an exploratory study of white and ethnic minority employees using the grounded theory approach, unpublished Masters thesis, School of Psychology, University of Leeds.

Miller, P. and Sperry, L. (1987) The socialisation of anger and aggression, *Merill Palmer Quarterly*, 33, 1–31.

Miller, S.M., Lack, E.R. and Asroff, S. (1985) Preferences for control and the coronary prone behavior pattern: I'd rather do it myself, *Journal of Personality and Social Psychology*, 49, 492–499.

Monroe, R.R. (1974) Maturational lag in central nervous system development as a partial explanation of episodic violent behaviour. In J. deWit and W.W. Hartup (eds) *Determinants and Origins of Aggressive Behaviour*, The Hague: Mouton.

Moutier, C.Y. and Stein, M.B. (1999) The history, epidemiology, and differential diagnosis of social anxiety disorder, *Journal of Clinical Psychiatry*, 60, 4–8.

Murray, C.Y. and Stein, M.B. (1999) The history, epidemiology and differential diagnosis of social anxiety disorder, *Journal of Clinical Psychology*, 60, 4–8.

Mynard, H. and Joseph, S. (1997) Bully/victim problems and their association with Eysenck's personality dimensions in 8 to 13 year olds, *British Journal of Educational Psychology*, 67, 51–54.

Nader, K.O. and Fairbanks, L.A. (1994) The suppression of reexperiencing: impulse control and somatic symptoms in children following traumatic exposure. Special issue: War and stress in the Middle East, *Anxiety, Stress and Coping*, 7, 229–239.

Nay, W. R. (1979) *Multimethod Clinical Assessment*, New York: Gardner.

Neuman, J.H. and Baron, R.A. (1997) Aggression in the workplace. In R. Giacalone and J. Greenberg (eds) *Antisocial Behavior in Organizations*, Thousand Oaks, CA: Sage, pp. 37–67.

Neuman, J.H. and Baron, R.A. (1998) Workplace violence and workplace aggression: evidence concerning specific forms, potential causes, and preferred targets, *Journal of Management*, 24, 391–419.

Newman, C.J. (1976) Children of disaster: clinical observations at Buffalo Creek, *American Journal of Psychiatry*, 133, 306–312.

Niedl, K. (1996) Mobbing and well-being: economic and personnel development implications, *European Journal of Work and Organizational Psychology*, 5, 239–249.

Olafsen, R.N. and Viemero, V. (2000) Bully/victim problems and coping with stress in school among 10- to 12-year-old pupils in Aland, Finland, *Aggressive Behavior*, 26, 57–65.

Olweus, D. (1978) *Aggression in the Schools: Bullies and Whipping Boys*, Washington, DC: Hemisphere Press.

Olweus, D. (1980) Familial and temperamental determinants of aggressive behaviour in adolescent boys: a causal analysis, *Developmental Psychology*, 16, 644–660.

Olweus, D. (1989) Prevalence and incidence in the study of anti-social behavior: definitions and measurement. In M. Klein (ed.) *Cross-national Research in Self-reported Crime and Delinquency*, Dordrecht: Kluwer.

Olweus, D. (1993) *Bullying at School: What We Know and What We Can Do*, Oxford: Blackwell.

O'Moore, A.M., Kirkham, C. and Smith, M. (1997) Bullying in Irish schools: a nationwide study, *Irish Journal of Psychology*, 18, 141–169.

O'Moore, A.M., Seigne, E., McGuire, S. and Smith, M. (1998) Victims of bullying at work in Ireland, *Journal of Occupational Health and Safety*, 14, 569–574.

Osterman, M., Bjorkqvist, K., Largerspetz, K.M.J., Charpentier, S., Caprara, G.V. and Pastorelli, C. (1999) Locus of control and three types of aggression, *Aggressive Behavior*, 25, 61–65.

Otto, M.W. (1999) Cognitive-behavioral therapy for social anxiety: models, methods and outcome, *Journal of Clinical Psychiatry*, 60, 14–19.

Parens, H. (1979) *The Development of Aggression in Early Childhood*, New York: Jason Aronson.

Parke, R.D. and Slaby, R.G. (1983) The development of aggression. In P.H. Maissen, (ed.) *Handbook of Child Psychology* (4th edn) (Vol. 4), New York: Wiley, pp. 547–642.

Parker, G. (1983) *Parental Overprotection: A Risk Factor in Psychosocial Development*. New York: Grune and Stratton.

Parker, I. (1991) *Discourse Dynamics: Critical Analysis for Social and Individual Psychology*, London: Sage.

Pastorelli, C. (1999) Locus of control and three types of aggression, *Aggressive Behavior*, 25, 61–65.

Patterson, G.R. (1982) *Coercive Family Process*, Eugene, OR: Castilia.

Patterson, G.R. (1986) Maternal rejection: determinant or product of deviant clutch behaviour. In W. Hartup and K. Rubin (eds) *Relationships and Development*, Hillsdale, NJ: McGruner Hill.

Patterson, G.R., DeBaryshe, B.D. and Ramsey, E. (1989) A developmental perspective on antisocial behavior, *American Psychologist*, 44, 329–355.

Peneff, J. (1990) Myths in life stories. In R. Samuel and P. Thompson (eds) *The Myths We Live By*, London: Routledge.

Pepler, D., Craig, W., Zeigler, S. and Charach, A. (1993) A school-based anti-bullying intervention: preliminary evaluation. In D. Tattum (ed.) *Understanding and Managing Bullying*, Harlow: Longman, pp. 76–91.

Pettit, G.S., Harrist, A.W., Bates, J.E. and Dodge, K.A. (1991) Family interaction, social cognition and children's subsequent relations with peers at kindergarten, *Journal of Social and Personal Relationships*, 8, 393–402.

Phillips, K.A. (2000) Quality of life for patients with body dysmorphic disorder, *Journal of Nervous and Mental Disease*, 188, 170–175.

Phillips, K.A. and McElroy, S.L. (2000) Personality disorders and traits in patients with body dysmorphic disorder, *Comprehensive Psychiatry*, 41, 229–236.

Pikas, A. (1989) A pure concept of mobbing gives the best results for treatment, *School Psychology International*, 10, 95–104.

Pitts, J. and Smith, P.K. (1994) *Preventing School Bullying*, London: Home Office Police Research Group.

Plaud, J.J. and Newberry, D.E. (1996) Rule-governed behavior and pedophilia, *Sexual Abuse: A Journal of Research and Treatment*, 8, 143–151.

Plaud, J.J. and Plaud, D.M. (1998) Clinical behaviour therapy and the experimental analysis of behavior, *Journal of Clinical Psychology*, 54, 905–921.

Plomin, R. and Daniels, D. (1986) Genetics and shyness. In W.H. Jones, J.M. Check and S.R. Broggs (eds) *Shyness: Perspectives on Research and Treatment*, New York: Plenum.

Power, T. and Chapieski, M. (1986) Childrearing and impulse control in toddlers: a naturalistic investigation, *Developmental Psychology*, 22, 271–275.

Premack, D. and Woodruff, G. (1978) Does the chimpanzee have a theory of mind? *Behavioral and Brain Sciences*, 4, 515–526.

Pynoos, R.S. and Eth, S. (1985) Children traumatised by witnessing acts of personal violence: homicide, rape and suicide behaviour. In S. Eth and R.S. Pynoos (eds) *Posttraumatic Stress Disorder in Children*, Washington, DC: American Psychiatric Press.

Pynoos, R.S., Frederick, C., Nader, K. and Arroyo, W. (1987) Life threat and posttraumatic stress in school-age children, *Archives of General Psychiatry*, 44, 1057–1063.

Quine, L. (1999) Workplace bullying in the NHS community trust: staff questionnaire survey, *British Medical Journal*, 318, 228–232.

Ramage, R. (1996) *New Law Journal*, 1 November 1996.

Ramsey, P. (1987) Possession episodes in young children's social interactions, *Journal of Genetic Psychology*, 148, 315–324.

Randall, P.E. (1993) Tackling aggressive behaviour in the under-fives, *Journal of Family Health Care*, 3, 178–180.

Randall, P.E. (1994) The adult bullies, *Yorkshire on Sunday*, August 1994.

Randall, P.E. (1995) A factor study of the attitudes of children to victims in a high risk area, *Educational Psychology*, 11(3), 22–27.

Randall, P.E. (1996) *A Community Approach to Bullying*, Stoke-on-Trent: Trentham Books.

Randall, P.E. (1997a) *Adult Bullying: Victims and Perpetrators*, London: Routledge.

Randall, P.E. (1997b) Pre-school routes to bullying. In D. Tattum and G. Herbert (eds) *Bullying: Home, School and Community*, London: Routledge.

Randall, P.E. (1998) Aggression at school, post-traumatic stress disorder and children's peer relations. In P.T. Slee and K. Rigby *Children's Peer Relations: Current Issues and Future Directions*, London: Routledge.

Randall, P.E. and Donohue, M. (1993) Tackling bullying as a community, *Child Education*, 70, 78–80.

Randall, P.E. and Parker, J. (2000) Adult bullying: working with victims. In H. Kemshall and J. Pritchard (eds) *Good Practice in Working with Victims of Violence*, London: Jessica Kingsley.

Raphael, B., Lundin, T. and Weisaeth, L. (1989) A research method for the study of psychological and psychiatric aspects of disaster, *Acta Psychiatrica Scandinavia*, 80, 353.

Raven, B.H. (1992) A power interactional model of interpersonal influence, *Journal of Social behavior and Personality*, 7, 217–224.

Rayner, C. (1997) Incidence of workplace bullying, *Journal of Community and Applied Social Psychology*, 7, 199–208.

Rayner, C., Sheehan, M. and Barker, M. (1999) Theoretical approaches to the study of bullying at work, *International Journal of Manpower*, 20, 11–15.

Rigby, K. (1994) Psychological functioning in families of Australian adolescent school children involved in bully/victim problems, *Journal of Family Therapy*, 16, 173–187.

Rigby, K. (1997) What children tell us about bullying in schools, *Child Australia*, 22, 28–34.

Rigby, K. and Slee, P.T. (1999a) Effects of parenting on the peer relations of Australian adolescents, *Journal of Social Psychology*, 139, 387–388.

Rigby, K. and Slee, P.T. (1999b) Suicidal intention among adolescent children, *Suicide and Life Threatening Behaviour*, 2, 119–130.

Rigby, K., Slee, P.T. and Cunningham, R. (1999) Effects of parenting on the peer relations of Australian adolescents, *Journal of Social Psychology*, 139, 387–388.

Riley, W.T. and Treiber, F.A. (1989) The validity of self-report anger and hostility measures, *Journal of Clinical Psychology*, 45, 397–404.

Rodgers, A.V. (1993) The assessment of variables related to the parenting behaviour of mothers with young children, *Child and Youth Services Review*, 15(5), 385–402.

Rogers, R.W. (1980) Expressions of aggression: aggression-inhibiting effects of anonymity to authority and threatened retaliation, *Personality and Social Psychology Bulletin*, 6, 315–320.

Rubin, K.H. (1985) Socially withdrawn children: an 'at risk' population? In B.H. Schneider, K.H. Rubin and J.E. Ledingham (eds) *Peer Relationships and Social Skills in Childhood: Issues in Assessment and Training*, New York: Springer-Verlag.

Rubin, K.H., Chen, X. and Hymel, S. (1993) The socio-emotional characteristics of extremely aggressive and extremely withdrawn children, *Merill Palmer Quarterly*, 39, 518–534.

Rubin, K.H., Daniels-Beirness, T. and Bream, L. (1984) Social isolation and social problem solving: a longitudinal study, *Journal of Consulting and Clinical Psychology*, 52, 17–25.

Rubin, K.H. and Krasnor, L.R. (1986) Social cognitive and social behavioral perspectives on problem-solving. In M. Perlmutter (ed.) *Minnesota Symposia on Child Psychology* (Vol. 18), Hillsdale, NJ: Lawrence Erlbaum, pp. 1–68.

Rubin, K.H. and Mills, R.S.L. (1988) The many faces of social-isolation in childhood, *Journal of Consulting and Clinical Psychology*, 56, 916–924.

Rubin, K.H. and Mills, S.L. (1992) Parents' thoughts about children's socially adaptive and maladaptive behaviours: stability, change and individual differences. In I. Sigel, J. Goodnow and A.W. McGullicuddy-deLisi (eds) *Parental Belief Systems*, Hillsdale NJ: Lawrence Erlbaum.

Rubin, K.H., Mills, R.S.L. and Rose-Krasnor, L. (1989) Maternal beliefs and children's social competence. In B. Schneider, G. Attili, J. Nadel and R. Weissberg (eds) *Social Competence in Developmental Perspective*, Netherlands: Kluwer International Publishers.

Russell, G. (1987) *Notes on Eliciting and Recording Clinical Information in Psychiatric Patients* (2nd edn), Oxford: Oxford University Press.

Schachter, S. and Singer, J. (1962) Cognitive, social and physiological determinants of emotional state, *Psychological Review*, 69, 379–399.

Schuckit, M.A. and Hesselbrock, V. (1994) Alcohol dependence and anxiety disorders: what is the relationship? *American Journal of Psychiatry*, 151, 1723–1734.

Schwartz, D., Dodge, K.A. and Coie, J.D. (1993) The emergence of chronic peer victimization in boys' playgroups, *Child Development*, 64, 1755–1772.

Schwartz, D., Dodge, K.A., Pettit, G.S. and Bates, J.E. (1997) The early socialization of the aggressive victims of bullying, *Child Development*, 68, 665–675.

Seigne, E. (1998) Bullying at work in Ireland. In *Bullying at Work*, 1998 conference proceedings, Stafford: The Andrea Adams Trust, Staffordshire University Business School.

Sharp, S. and Thompson, D. (1992) Sources of stress: a contrast between pupil perspectives and pastoral teachers' perspectives, *School Psychology International*, 13, 229–242.

Sheehan, M. (1998) Restructuring: rhetoric versus reality. In P. McCarthy, P.M. Sheehan, S. Wilkie and W. Wilkie (eds) *Bullying: Causes, Costs and Cures*, Nathan: Beyond Bullying Association.

Siann, G. (1985) *Accounting for Human Aggression: Perspectives on Aggression and Violence*, Boston, MA: Allen and Unwin.

Sigel, I.E. (1982) The relationship between parental distancing strategies and the child's cognitive behaviour. In L.M. Lavsa and I.E. Sigel (eds) *Families as Learning Environments for their Children*, New York: Plenum.

Slee, P.T. and Rigby, K. (1993) The relationship of Eysenck's personality factors and self-esteem to bully–victim behaviour in Australian schoolboys, *Personality and Individual Differences*, 14, 371–373.

Smith, J. (1996) Beyond the divide between cognition and discourse: using interpretative phenomenological analysis in health psychology, *Psychology and Health*, 11, 261–271.

Smith, M.L., Carayon, P., Sanders, K.L., Lim, S.Y. and LeGrande, D. (1992) Employee stress and health complaints in jobs with and without electronic performance monitoring, *Applied Ergonomics*, 23, 17–28.

Smith, P.K. and Brain, P. (2000) Bullying in schools: lessons from two decades of research, *Aggressive Behavior*, 26, 1–9.

Smith, P.K. and Myron-Wilson, R. (1998) Parenting and school bullying, *Clinical Child Psychology and Psychiatry*, 3, 405–417.

Smith, P.K. and Sharp, S. (1994) *School Bullying*, London: Routledge.

Snyder, M., and Gangestad, S. (1986) On the nature of self-monitoring: matters of assessment, matters of validity, *Journal of Personality and Social Psychology*, 5, 125–139.

Spielberger, C.D., Jacobs, G., Russell, S. and Crane, R. (1983) Assessment of anger: the Stait-Trait Anger Scale. In J.N. Butcher and C.D. Spielberger (eds) *Advances in Personality Assessment* (Vol. 2), Hillsdale, NJ: Lawrence Erlbaum.

Sroufe, L.A. (1988) The role of infant–caregiver attachment in development. In J. Belsky and T. Nezworski (eds) *Clinical Implications of Attachment*, Hillsdale, NJ: Lawrence Erlbaum.

Staddon, J.E.R. (1983) *Adaptive Behavior and Learning*, Cambridge: Cambridge University Press.

Steerneman, P., Jackson, S., Pelzer, H. and Muris, P. (1996) Children with social handicaps: an intervention programme using a theory of mind approach, *Clinical Child Psychology and Psychiatry*, 1, 2.

Stein, M.B., McQuaid, J.R., Laffaye, C. and McCahill, M.E. (1999) Social phobia in the primary care medical setting, *Journal of Family Practice*, 48, 514–519.

Steinberg, L., Lamborn, S.D., Dornbusch, S.M. and Darling, N. (1992) Impact of parenting practices on adolescent achievement: authoritative parenting, school involvement and encouragement to succeed, *Child Development*, 63, 1266–1281.

Stern, D. (1985) *The Interpersonal World of the Infant*, New York: Basic Books.

Stewart, S.L. and Rubin, K.H. (1995) The social problem-solving skills of anxious-withdrawn children, *Development and Psychopathology*, 7, 323–336.

Storms, P.L. and Spector, P.E. (1987) Relationships of organizational frustration with reported behavioral reactions: the moderating effect of locus of control, *Journal of Occupational Psychology*, 60, 227–234.

Sutton, J., Smith, P.K. and Swettenham, J. (1999) Bullying and 'theory of mind': a critique of the 'social skills deficit' view of anti-social behaviour, *Social Development*, 8, 117–125.

Szegal, B. (1985) Stages in the development of aggressive behaviours in early childhood, *Aggressive Behavior*, 11, 315–321.

Tedeschi, J.T. (1983) Social influence theory and aggression. In R.G. Green and E. Donnerstein (eds) *Aggression – Theoretical and Empirical Reviews, Volume 1 – Theoretical and Methodological Issues*, New York: Academy Press, pp. 77–101.

Terr, L.C. (1979) Children of Chowchilla: study of psychic trauma, *Psychoanalytic Study of the Child*, 34, 547–623.

Terr, L.C. (1989) Treating psychic trauma in children: a preliminary discussion, *Journal of Traumatic Stress*, 2, 3–20.

Terr, L.C. (1995) Childhood traumas: an outline and overview. In G.S. Everly and J.M. Lating (eds) *Psychotraumatology*, New York: Plenum, pp. 301–320.

Trades Union Congress (1998) *No Excuse: Beat Bullying at Work: A Guide for Trade Union Representatives and Personnel Managers*, London: TUC.

Tremblay, R.E. (2000) The development of aggressive behaviour during childhood, *International Journal of Behavioural Development*, 24, 129–141.

Tronick, E.Z. (1989) Emotions and emotional communication in infants, *American Psychologist*, 44, 112–119.

Troy, M. and Sroufe, L.A. (1987) Victimization among preschoolers: role of attachment relationship history, *Journal of the American Academy of Child and Adolescent Psychiatry*, 26, 166–172.

Tsui, A.S., Egan, T.D. and O'Reilly, C.A. (1994) Being different: relational demography and organizational attachment, *Administrative Science Quarterly*, 37, 549–579.

Vartia, M. (1996) The sources of bullying – psychological work environment and organizational climate, *European Journal of Work and Organizational Psychology*, 5, 203–214.

Vaughn, B., Kopp, C. and Kurakow, J. (1984) The emergence and consolidation of self control from 18 to 30 months of age: normative trends and individual differences, *Child Development*, 55, 990–1004.

Weaver, A.A.F. (2000) Can post-traumatic stress disorder be diagnosed in adolescence without a catastrophic stressor? A case report, *Clinical Child Psychology and Psychiatry*, 5, 7–83.

Weisfeld, G.E. (1994) Aggression and dominance in the social world of boys. In J. Archer (ed.), *Male Violence*, London: Routledge.

Weiss, B., Dodge, K.A., Bates, J.E. and Pettit, G.S. (1992) Some consequences of early harsh discipline: child aggression and maladaptive information processing, *Child Development*, 63, 1321–1335.

Werner, P.D., Rose, T.L., Yesavage, J.A. and Seeman, K. (1984) Psychiatrists' judgments of dangerousness in patients on an acute care unit, *American Journal of Psychiatry*, 141, 263–266.

Worchel, S. and Teddlie, C. (1976) The experience of crowding: a two factor theory, *Journal of Personality and Social Psychology*, 34, 30–40.

Young, J.E. (1989) *Schema-focused Cognitive Therapy for Personality Disorders and Difficult Patients*, Sarasota, FL: Professional Resource Exchange.

Zapf, D. (1999) Organisational, work group related and personal causes of mobbing/bullying at work, *International Journal of Manpower*, 20, 70–85.

Zapf, D., Knorz, C. and Kulla, M. (1996) On the relationship between mobbing factors, and job content, social work environment and health outcomes, *European Journal of Work and Organizational Psychology*, 5, 215–237.

Zillmann, D. (1971) Excitation transfer in communication-mediated aggressive behaviour, *Journal of Experimental and Social Psychology*, 7, 419–434.

Zillmann, D. (1996) Anger. In *Encyclopedia of Mental Health*, New York: Harcourt Brace.

Zimbardo, P.G. (1970) The human choice: individuation, reason and order versus deindividuation, impulse and chaos. In W.J. Arnold and D. Levine (eds) *Nebraska Symposium on Motivation*, Lincoln, NB: University of Nebraska Press.

Index